Praise for *Trauma Healing in the Yoga Zone*

In Trauma Healing in the Yoga Zone *Joann Lutz transforms yoga practices into a neurobiological based therapeutic strategy that facilitates and optimizes health through enhanced autonomic regulation. This model, which she names Nervous System-Informed, Trauma-Sensitive Yoga (NITYA), is the product of an insightful consilience of ancient traditions with contemporary neuroscience. Embracing the model will lead to deeper understanding of the wisdom embedded in yoga and the powerful neurophysiological impact it may have on rehabilitating mental and physical health.*

Stephen W. Porges, PhD: Distinguished University Scientist, Kinsey Institute, Indiana University, Bloomington; Professor, Department of Psychiatry, University of North Carolina at Chapel Hill

In Trauma Healing in the Yoga Zone, *Joann Lutz combines ancient wisdom from yoga with a scientifically informed therapeutic approach for safe and effective trauma resolution. Compulsory reading for anyone interested in healing trauma through neuroscience blended with compassion!*

Shirley Telles, MBBS PhD: Director, Patanjali Research Foundation

With over 5% of the population experiencing trauma that leads to clinically significant post-traumatic stress disorder, its prevalence is becoming more recognized in society. Neuroscientific research is revealing that this condition is a mind-body disorder, and yet conventional treatments such as psychotherapy focus on cognitive processes and have been only partially effective. This book comprehensively describes the theory and application of yoga as a mind-body intervention for trauma. It is a welcome contribution to the growing field of trauma-sensitive yoga that will be of significant use to both patients and therapists.

Sat Bir Singh Khalsa, PhD: Assistant Professor of Medicine, Harvard Medical School; Editor in Chief, International Journal of Yoga Therapy; Editor, The Principles and Practice of Yoga in Health Care

An innovative approach to healing trauma.

Dean Ornish, MD: Author of *"UnDo It!"*; Founder and President, Preventive Medicine Research Institute; Clinical Professor of Medicine, UCSF

Joann Lutz offers an in-depth exploration of accessible methods to address the complexity of trauma through comprehensive understandings of the nervous system and yoga philosophy and practices. Her writing supports the reader in reflecting upon the many nuances of applying these theories and practices for trauma sensitivity. This book is a valuable resource to anyone wanting to learn more about how yoga can safely and effectively benefit people who have experienced trauma.

Marlysa Sullivan, DPT, C-IAYT: Author of Understanding Yoga Therapy: Applied Philosophy and Science for Wellbeing

Joann has wondrously woven together multiple disparate models of how yoga affects the post-traumatic nervous system, to enhance our understanding and utilization of these practices. This work will be a cherished contribution to the growing body of work on these ever evolving theories.

Jonathan Rosenthal, MD: Resident Physician, Neurology, NYU School of Medicine; www.neuroyoganyc.com; www.jonathanrosenthalmd.com

These days, when I teach, I hear a common question from yoga therapy students: What's the evidence for this? Trauma Healing in the Yoga Zone is the perfect place to send them for answers, and to look them up myself! Joann Lutz does a remarkable job of linking specific practices to their effects on the autonomic nervous system. Each recommended practice is backed up by scientific evidence or, if the data is not yet available, current scientific theory. The research behind why and how yoga can help trauma survivors heal is invaluable for yoga therapists and mental health practitioners. I will be referencing this rich compendium of research and practice for years to come!

Amy Weintraub, MFA, C-IAYT, YACEP: Author of *Yoga Skills for Therapists, Yoga for Depression*, and the card deck, Yoga for Your Mood

Trauma Healing in the Yoga Zone *is the book that all yoga teachers and yoga therapists will benefit from reading. It is the perfect bridge between the teachings of yoga, modern allopathic medicine, and the psychology of healing trauma. The book explains in detail how the nervous system functions when it is healthy vs dysregulated, and how to bring it back to balance using the tools of yoga. I will be recommending it to all of my students and colleagues!*

Amy Wheeler, PhD (Southern California): Former President of the International Association of Yoga Therapists (2018–2020); www.amywheeler.com

As a certified yoga therapist working with clients who suffer, it is evident how trauma affects the body and mind as one. Trauma Healing in the Yoga Zone offers an extensive wealth of comprehensive, evidence-based knowledge to yoga therapists, to enrich their work, and to mental health professionals, to enhance their work with accessible yogic practices. This book is of great value for training as well as practice in both professions.

Helene Couvrette, C-IAYT, E-RYT500: President MISTY – Montreal International Symposium on Therapeutic Yoga; Founder H~OM Yoga; www.homyogacenter.com

Trauma Healing in the Yoga Zone

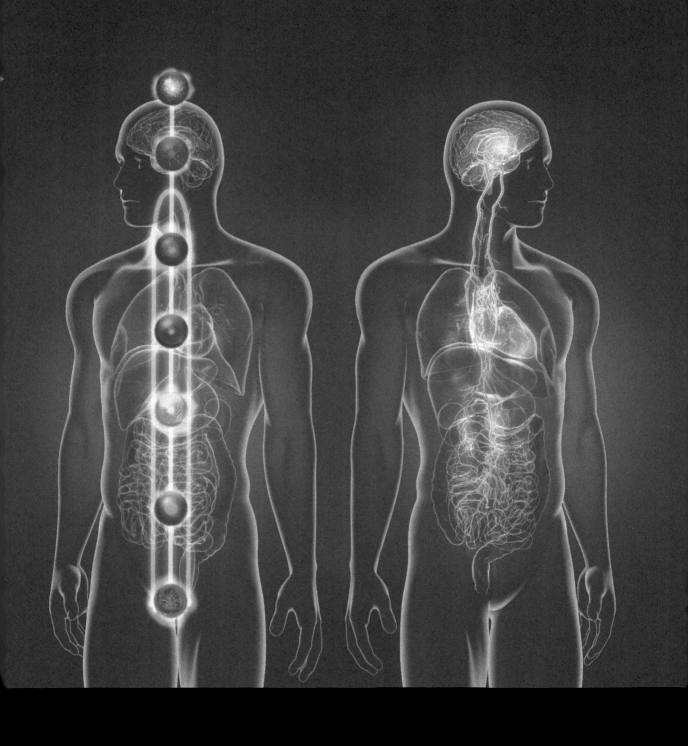

Trauma Healing in the Yoga Zone

A guide for mental health professionals
and yoga therapists and teachers

Joann Lutz

Forewords
Arielle Schwartz
Sandra McLanahan

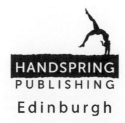

HANDSPRING
PUBLISHING
Edinburgh

HANDSPRING PUBLISHING LIMITED
The Old Manse, Fountainhall, Pencaitland, East Lothian EH34 5EY, Scotland
Tel: +44 1875 341 859
Website: www.handspringpublishing.com

First published 2021 in the United Kingdom by Handspring Publishing Limited
Copyright © Handspring Publishing Limited 2021

4

ISBN 978-1-912085-07-1
ISBN (Kindle eBook) 978-1-912085-08-8

British Library Cataloguing in Publication Data
A catalogue record for this book is available from the British Library
Library of Congress Cataloging in Publication Data
A catalog record for this book is available from the Library of Congress

Eye movement script on pages 34–35 and 116–117 includes material from *Accessing the Healing Power of the Vagus Nerve: Self-Help Exercises for Anxiety, Depression, Trauma, and Autism* by Stanley Rosenberg, published by North Atlantic Books, copyright © 2017 by Stanley Rosenberg. Reprinted by permission of North Atlantic Books.

All the photos of Deluxey Puvanasingam were taken by Richard Getler.

Commissioning Editor Sarena Wolfaard
Project Manager Morven Dean
Copy Editor Kathryn Mason Pak
Designer Bruce Hogarth
Indexer Aptara, India
Typesetter DSM, India
Printer CPI Group (UK) Ltd, Croydon, CR0 4YY
Book printed in Minion Pro Regular 12/13.5pt

The
Publisher's
policy is to use
paper manufactured
from sustainable forests

This book is dedicated to my late parents, Elwood and Isobel Tuvman Lutz, for their love and support; to all of my ancestors, who struggled to survive and nurture life; and to courageous trauma survivors, worldwide, who have spoken out about their abuse.

CONTENTS

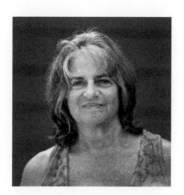

Joann Lutz MSW, LICSW, C-IAYT, E-RYT

Joann, psychotherapist and yoga therapist/teacher, is a pioneer in the application of trauma-sensitive yoga to mental health care. She developed and continues to teach the Nervous System-Informed, Trauma-Sensitive Yoga model of care (NITYA), which incorporates classical yoga, neuroscience research, and somatic psychotherapy. This work rests on her background in Integral Yoga®, Somatic Experiencing®, Ayurvedic Yoga Therapy, EMDR, and Psychosynthesis.

She is the author of the NASW-MA CE course "Bringing Yoga into Social Work Practice" and the paper, "Classical Yoga Postures as a Psychotherapeutic Intervention for Autonomic Nervous System Regulation," published in the Proceedings of the Yoga and Psyche Conference, 2014 (Newcastle upon Tyne: Cambridge Scholars; 2016). Her website is www.yogainpsychotherapy.com.

In the process of writing this book, searching for the elements of yoga which had resulted in so much healing for myself, and for so many others, I became a something of a "yoga sleuth." My first clue was the emphasis on the regulating effect of working with the autonomic nervous system for trauma healing, as presented in the Somatic Experiencing® (SE™) training. That turned out to be the key which opened the first door: the realization that many of yoga's physical postures, and particularly those I was most familiar with, as taught in the Integral Yoga® Institute's classes, were organized around balancing the branches of that system. Further examination of that discovery, through practice and a review of the research, has confirmed it.

The next key was the assertion in many yoga traditions that the breathing practices were yoga's most powerful tool. Further study of those practices revealed striking correspondences between the subtle nervous system, as it was described in yogic texts, and the action of the autonomic nervous system. The plot was deepening.

The key which opened the third door was my discovery of polyvagal theory, developed by Dr Stephen Porges, which emphasized the healing effect on the nervous system of the experience of safety. The word "safety" described my own experience of practicing in a quiet, physically secure yoga studio, presided over by a compassionate and focused, but relaxed, instructor, and guided by a centuries-old philosophy of non-injury to self and others.

Finally, approaching door number four, was a realization that the gunas, described in the Bhagavad Gita as the basic qualities of all matter, seemed to correspond to the action of the autonomic nervous system. As I was pondering the similarities of these disparate systems, I discovered an article with physical therapist and yoga therapist Marlysa Sullivan as the lead researcher, and listing Dr Stephen Porges as one of the contributors (Sullivan et al., 2018), which postulated exactly that. This gave an added impetus to my searches in this area and to my learning, as reflected in this book.

I hope that you and your clients will benefit from the discoveries which are presented in this book, and that, as a result, we will all make our world a safer place.

Joann Lutz
Florence, Massachusetts, USA
April 2021

Joann and I met in quite a serendipitous manner several years ago at a conference for the United States Association of Body Psychotherapy (USABP). We had each arrived early in preparation for our presentations and were seated outdoors on the sunny, California campus of Pacifica University. We quickly learned of our shared interest in therapeutic yoga as an adjunct to therapy and, more specifically, for the treatment of trauma. We spent the afternoon engaged in lively conversation in which we also learned of our mutual appreciation for polyvagal theory as a foundation for our work. This initial conversation has evolved into a lasting connection sparked by our passion for the unique blend of neuroscience, psychology, and spirituality that lives at the intersection of yoga and psychotherapy.

In our modern world, the ancient practices of meditation and yoga are increasingly being integrated into psychotherapy as a complementary approach to traditional therapies. Clients are seeking out mindfulness-based modalities of treatment as part of a larger movement that is reducing stigma around mental health concerns. Research suggests that most people will experience at least one traumatic event in their lifetime and that exposure to multiple traumatic events is the norm (Kilpatrick at al., 2013). With this knowledge, we are invited to turn toward our own life challenges with greater acceptance and with the knowledge that we are not alone. Simply put, post-traumatic stress is becoming increasingly understood, depathologized, and normalized.

Psychotherapy is often sought out to reduce the emotional and physiological symptoms of post-traumatic stress. It is quite normal to experience feelings of agitation, panic, or irritability and somatic symptoms of shakiness, nausea, or dizziness. Moreover, when traumatic events are ongoing or repeated we might have predominant feelings of helplessness and powerlessness which can correspond with feeling physiologically collapsed, emotionally numb, or disconnected from our body. These emotions and sensations can feel confusing, overwhelming, or frightening when we do not have sufficient support. Traditional therapies often focus on the narrative related to traumatic events but fail to teach clients how to work with or through their somatic distress that is the result of a dysregulated autonomic nervous system. In order to reduce physiological symptoms, clients are frequently referred for psychiatric medications which may offer temporary reprieve from distress, but risk side effects or concerns about long-term dependency. Most importantly, these approaches to care often mask symptoms but fail to address the underlying cause.

The emergence of therapeutic yoga offers a much needed natural approach to trauma recovery (van der Kolk et al., 2014). Here, we discover tools to help clients address the physiological effects of trauma through gentle breath and movement practices that regulate the autonomic nervous system from the inside out (Tyagi & Cohen, 2016). Moreover, yogic philosophy invites a softening of aggressive thoughts or actions such as self-criticism or self-harming behaviors. In addition to helping clients manage the distress of their symptoms, yoga offers an opportunity to attend to and possibly resolve the underlying nervous system dysregulation.

Many therapists desire to bring yoga into their clinical work but don't know where to start. Others may bring to their clients yoga postures or breath practices without sufficient awareness of the possible contraindications of these interventions. This book, *Trauma Healing in the Yoga Zone*, provides a structure that will undoubtedly guide clinicians to safely and seamlessly integrate yogic practices into psychotherapy sessions. Joann's NITYA program

FOREWORD *continued*

offers accessible chair yoga postures and wisely chosen breath practices that increase the reach of what may otherwise feel like an elusive practice. Her model of therapeutic yoga is grounded in modern neuroscience and traditional yogic wisdom.

I have been teaching yoga for over twenty-five years and I am pleased to say that I personally took away from this book an enhanced understanding of how pranayama can help us to balance the autonomic nervous system. For example, the commonly taught practice of Ujjayi pranayama is often described as having a calming effect on the nervous system; however, Joann cautions her readers that this simple practice can lead to increased agitation of the sympathetic nervous system due to constriction in the throat. Instead, she provides a scientifically grounded basis for her recommendations to teach the three-part deep breath (deerga swasam), alternate nostril breathing (nadi shodhana), and honeybee (brahmari) pranayama.

Drawing from her training in Somatic Experiencing® and polyvagal theory, Joann describes the cascade of defensive physiological responses that underlie the suffering experienced by trauma survivors. Moreover, she guides a process of releasing the imprints that linger as arousal states in the nervous system and sensations in the body. She helps us trust that we can find freedom in the body – at a safe pace tailored to the individual. She reminds us that trauma is not a life sentence. Most importantly, this book reads like a gift from Joann's deeply spiritual heart. She instills a sense of hope and encouragement that we can, in time, release the burden of trauma and heal.

Arielle Schwartz, PhD
Clinical Psychologist,
Certified Kripalu Yoga Teacher
Author of *The Complex PTSD Workbook* and
The Post-Traumatic Growth Guidebook
Boulder, Colorado, USA
February 2021

References

Kilpatrick, D.G., Resnick, H.S., Milanak, M.E., Miller, M.W., Keyes, K.M., Friedman, M.J. (2013) National estimates of exposure to traumatic events and PTSD prevalence using DSM-IV and DSM-5 criteria. *Journal Traumatic Stress*, 26: 537–47.

Tyagi, A., & Cohen, M. (2016) Yoga and heart rate variability: A comprehensive review of the literature. *International Journal of Yoga*, 9(2): 97–113.

van der Kolk, B.A., Stone, L., West, J., Rhodes, A., Emerson, D., Suvak, M., & Spinazzola, J. (2014) Yoga as an adjunctive treatment for posttraumatic stress disorder: A randomized controlled trial. *Journal of Clinical Psychiatry*, 75(6): e559–e565.

FOREWORD by Sandra McLanahan

Joann Lutz is a creative and insightful author who has developed this yoga-based approach to trauma healing from her extensive experience as a yoga practitioner, psychotherapist, and researcher. I know Joann as a sincere student of Integral Yoga®, which she has studied for the past fifty years.

In *Trauma Healing in the Yoga Zone* Joann has written a book which is of value to everyone who works with individuals who have experienced psychological trauma and related conditions. It breaks new ground, particularly for mental health providers, providing a depth of understanding of the therapeutic value of yoga and its practical applications, as well as recent contributions from the field of neuroscience.

The negative effects of trauma and stress are especially difficult, creating tension, anxiety, depression, and other acutely painful and chronically disabling diseases. Research has shown that a physiological approach to healing trauma-related conditions complements the well-established cognitive and affective approaches of traditional psychotherapy. Joann's approach can therefore be seen as a bridge between the field of psychotherapy and the practice of lifestyle medicine.

When cued to the nervous-system state of the client, the tools of yoga – particularly the postures, breathing practices, and relaxation techniques – can help to create the conditions of calm within. Even one session has been documented to change the body's physiology, including hormone and fatigue levels, because of yoga's powerful ability to re-balance the sympathetic and parasympathetic branches of the autonomic nervous system. It is certainly hopeful that yoga research is burgeoning, and that this ancient discipline being recognized for its many contributions to mental health maintenance in the complex world of the twenty-first century. *Trauma Healing in the Yoga Zone* could be seen as a primer for the synthesis of this ancient discipline and the current, scientifically based advances in mental health care.

Sandra McLanahan, MD
Past Director, Stress Management Training,
Preventive Medicine Research Institute,
Sausalito, California, USA
Co-author of *Surgery and Its Alternatives*
Contributor to *Dr. Yoga* and *After Cancer Care*
Yogaville, Buckingham, Virginia, USA
February 2021

ACKNOWLEDGMENTS

I would like to acknowledge the invaluable patience and kindness I received from Sarena Wolfaard, Commissioning Editor, Handspring Publishing, as well as my Handspring copyeditor, Kathryn Mason Pak, and Project Manager Morven Dean. Others who helped me tremendously are Sandra McLanahan, Kelly Birch, and Marlena Merrin, editors; Swami Dharmananda of the Sivananda Yoga Farm, who recorded the workshop presentation which became the basis for the book; and Claudia Zuniga, transcriptionist: thank you! I am also grateful for the many yoga and mental health professionals who guided me along the way. Among them are Shirley Telles, Marc Halpern, Steven Hoskinson, Dave Berger, Stephen Porges, Sat Bir Khalsa, Catherine Hondorp, Beth Dennison, Peter Payne, Becky Carroll, Suzanne Ludlum, Marlysa Sullivan, Alisa Wright Tanny, Mariana Caplan, Livia Budrys, Inge Senglemann, Barbara Kaplan, Nina Goradia, Deb Dana, Sally Roach, models Deluxey Puvanasingam and Stephen O'Neill, and photographer Richard Getler. I apologize to anyone who may have helped me with the book during the past five years, whom I forgot to mention.

Photographs by Richard Getler and Joann Lutz.

The case vignettes presented in the book are a composite of cases, reconfigured for their educational value.

Joann Lutz
Florence, Massachusetts, USA

INTRODUCTION

I have long been an observer of human behavior. One of my most memorable observations came when I was in high school. I noticed that one of my friends could lie on the couch, very relaxed, for hours, and then jump up and be instantly mobilized for action when the situation required it. She then could easily return to her resting state, unperturbed. The dynamic shift between her resting and active state struck me as remarkable. Later in life, I realized that I had witnessed something rare: a human being with a flexible, responsive autonomic nervous system (ANS)! This behavior contrasts with the individual with the dysregulated ANS, who may not be able to be assertive when the situation calls for it; to relax when there is no stressor; or, in severe cases, to perform the necessary tasks of daily life.

This observation hit home when, after a turbulent time in college in the 1960s, I came home with a major depression. I took what was offered by the psychiatry profession at the time, which was talk therapy and medication, but it was the discovery of yoga that gave me the strongest lifeline. My extended hatha yoga sessions every morning gave my life structure and purpose, enhanced my physical health, and calmed my mind. Little did I know that yoga was also regulating my ANS, which had derailed during those stressful years.

In addition, the books I read on yoga philosophy and history provided a glimpse into the wisdom of an ancient, nature-based culture. I took those gifts, too: a healthier diet, and a more fluid way to move, to breathe, and to think. My recovery was rapid and, it seems, permanent. As I recovered, I made a commitment to myself to do what I could to help individuals who found themselves in similar situations. This commitment has been the basis of my career, and of this book.

The psychotherapy profession has moved far and fast since then. Some benchmarks of its forward movement include the diagnosis of post-traumatic stress disorder (PTSD), introduced into the Diagnostic and Statistical Manual of Mental Disorders (known as the DSM) in 1980; the development of body-oriented therapy techniques by many pioneers in the 1970s and 1980s; the founding of the International Association of Yoga Therapists in 1989; and the introduction of trauma-sensitive yoga to the yoga and mental health fields in the early 2000s by Bessel van der Kolk, MD and his associates.

It has become clear to me that nervous system dysregulation is one of the defining characteristics of unhealed psychological trauma. The ANS becomes dysregulated when the individual is overwhelmed by a threatening situation, and is immobilized when a safe resolution, or an escape, is blocked. In those moments, it responds by either shifting into overdrive, starting to shut down, or both, simultaneously. When that happens, the system loses its ability to respond flexibly and appropriately to the situation at hand, either temporarily or for the long term.

This book presents a therapeutic approach, rooted in yoga practice, designed for trauma survivors and individuals with chronic anxiety and depression, which addresses nervous system dysregulation directly. I call it nervous system-informed, trauma-sensitive yoga (NITYA). NITYA is an integration of four domains: (1) classical Raja Yoga; (2) the basic anatomy and physiology of the human ANS; (3) neuropsychology research; and, to a lesser degree, (4) somatic psychotherapy. Polyvagal Theory, the work of Dr Stephen Porges, is a key to this integration.

The chapters which follow provide a foundation in these domains, as well as guidelines for their application as a coherent discipline. I see NITYA potentially as a healing experience in itself, and also as a preparation for deeper trauma work, using additional modalities.

One underlying principle of this approach is that somatic practices are crucial elements in healing psychological trauma. Another is that each individual dealing with these conditions is unique and has their own healing path. Each intervention is a mutual exploration, utilizing the therapist's knowledge, skill, and regulating presence in concert with the client's awareness and motivation.

It can be a big leap for a mental health professional to use a physically based discipline such as yoga and skillfully integrate it with psychotherapy, particularly if they are not trained in working with the body. It may be a similar challenge for some yoga therapists to use yoga in concert with psychotherapeutic approaches. NITYA aims to bridge these gaps.

Much of this book supports emerging collaborations, including psychotherapists who are also certified yoga teachers; occupational and physical therapists who incorporate yoga into their work; yoga teachers and body workers who are trauma-informed; and researchers who are penetrating human survival responses. It is compatible with many, if not all, approaches to psychotherapy and yoga therapy, such as Internal Family Systems, eye movement desensitization and reprocessing (EMDR), and Gestalt Therapy.

I am proud to help to usher in this new field of practice, and hope that you find value in it, and continue to develop it.

NOTE: Researchers have recommended the development of a yoga protocol that employs practices thought to impact specific physiological mechanisms (Uebelacker et al., 2016, p. 73). NITYA could provide a uniform methodology for research, which is currently hampered by the use of many different approaches to yoga practice, from different traditions, which typically fail to reference the underlying physiological processes which yoga may ameliorate.

Setting the stage for the study of nervous system-informed, trauma-sensitive yoga (NITYA)

A shift in perspective

Each time you take a deep breath, you are using your physiology to overcome the residual effects of some form of stress. When you relax into your chair, the release of muscular tension sends your autonomic nervous system a message of safety. When you move with awareness of your movement, you are inviting a present moment experience, which has the power to challenge your habitual patterns of perception. The science of yoga makes the most of these physiological regulating mechanisms, amplifying them for healing. These basic physiological processes are the basis for Nervous System-Informed, Trauma-Sensitive Yoga, the system which I describe in this book.

The following chart showing the Nervous System-Informed, Trauma-Sensitive Yoga (NITYA) Healing Model (Figure 1.1) summarizes this at a glance.

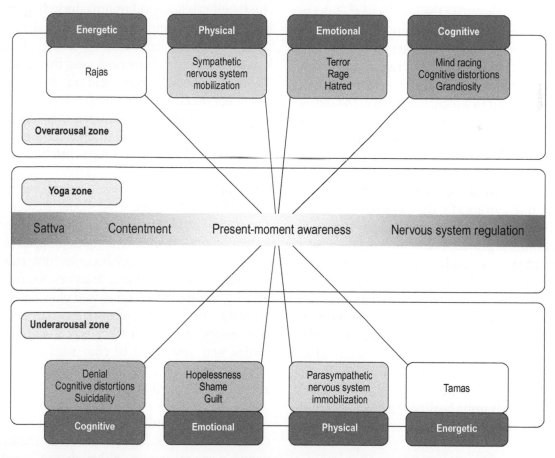

Figure 1.1 The Nervous System-Informed, Trauma-Sensitive Yoga (NITYA) Healing Model.

Chapter 1

You may first notice the four areas of therapeutic focus: physical, emotional, cognitive, and energetic. The chart presents the full range of the experience of each, along a continuum. They are superimposed upon a range of autonomic nervous system (ANS) states, from the most aroused to the most collapsed. For example, looking at the physical continuum, at the top end of the polarity, the sympathetic branch of the autonomic nervous system, which gives us energy and focus, is on overdrive, creating a set of distressing symptoms. At the bottom end, the parasympathetic branch of the nervous system (PNS), which normally functions to rejuvenate the body, will shut down, creating the opposite symptoms. The goal of the NITYA approach is to moderate the activation of both branches, so that they create healthy flow between them. When this happens, the activation will rise and fall in a regular pattern in the central area of the chart. The underlying concept for the diagram comes from Daniel Siegel, MD's concept of "the window of tolerance" (Siegel, 1999).

When applied to the trauma survivor, or anyone with a chronically dysregulated autonomic nervous system, the moderation of symptoms can produce a greater ability to tune into what is happening in one's body, and in the environment, moment to moment. In this regulated state, the individual can flexibly respond to the situation at hand. In this approach, it is the yogic interventions, adapted for trauma sensitivity and keyed to the individual's current autonomic state, which bring the system back into regulation. At that point, the regulated individual is in an optimal state for deep trauma healing. The yogic interventions, and their skillful use, are the substance of this book.

This approach offers a shift in focus in therapeutic work, from cognitive and affective to primarily physiological. Seen from this perspective, it becomes apparent that many of the symptoms of post-traumatic stress disorder (PTSD) are physiological as well as psychological. Examples are hypervigilance; an exaggerated startle response; problems with concentration; and sleep disturbances (American Psychiatric Association, 2017, p. 272).

Extensive data confirming the link between childhood trauma and adult disease support this shift. The Adverse Childhood Experiences (ACE) study found a consistent relationship between childhood psychological trauma, including physical, sexual, and emotional abuse, and the adult onset of ischemic heart disease, cancer, chronic lung disease, skeletal fractures, and liver disease. These are serious illnesses, and point to trauma as a major public health issue (Felitti et al., 1998). While the specific links between these medical conditions and childhood trauma have not yet been identified, the relationship is proven.

To understand and work comfortably with the NITYA model, the practitioner first needs a working knowledge of the autonomic nervous system, which influences emotions, thoughts, and subtle energies. As the work becomes more subtle, as it does in yogic breathing practices, the fourth polarity, the energetic, comes into play. The yoga tradition offers a comprehensive description of how energy operates in the physical and subtle bodies, and how it can be channeled for maximum health and nervous system regulation. This area will be explored in Chapter 2.

My own yoga teacher training, taken in 1980, did not include specific information on the autonomic nervous system, although the benefits of remaining alert and simultaneously relaxed as a result of yoga practice were emphasized.

While research results on the positive effect of certain yogic interventions on the physiology of trauma survivors support this link, I am aware of influential yoga schools that do not address trauma sensitivity as an essential element of the training. Yoga teacher training would benefit from a greater awareness of the effect of yoga practices on the autonomic nervous system, and on the link between nervous system regulation and trauma recovery. It is my belief that this book can help to bridge the two disciplines.

For all of these reasons, in this foundational chapter, I present information on the normal functioning of the human nervous system, and a detailed look at the negative effects of traumatic incidents on the ANS and the human body in general. The chapter also includes an introduction to polyvagal theory, interpersonal neurobiology, and neuroplasticity, which deepen the understanding of the physiological effects of trauma.

Overview of the nervous system

As has been mentioned, traditional psychotherapy training prepared the therapist to work with both thoughts and emotions, associated with the neo-cortex and limbic system, respectively (Stangor & Walinga, 2014). More recently, as a result of neuroimaging studies of the effects of trauma on the brain, attention has shifted to the functioning of the autonomic nervous system, located in the brain stem. The autonomic nervous system, has the important job of evaluating, regulating, and acting on internal sensations and external information in a coordinated way (Sullivan, 2020). Processes originating in the brain stem activate the mobilization responses of fight and flight and the various immobilization responses, as well as controlling many of the body processes which are not under our conscious control, such as digestion (OpenStax, 2016). This area of the brain is dysregulated in individuals with post-traumatic stress disorder (Thomas, 2018).

Understanding the autonomic nervous system, begins with an overview of the entire nervous system, which is made up of two parts: the central nervous system and the peripheral nervous system. The central nervous system includes the brain and spinal cord, which gather and process information. The peripheral nervous system transmits this information back and forth between the central nervous system and the rest of the body. It consists of the cranial nerves; the spinal nerves, along with their roots and branches; the peripheral nerves; and the neuromuscular junctions. The autonomic nervous system, along with the enteric nervous system, which enervates the digestive system (Furness et al., 2014), are both part of the peripheral nervous system.

Neurons that carry messages to the brain are labeled afferent. Afferent nerves function in both the somatic and autonomic nervous systems, relaying signals from the internal and external environments. Messages from the brain to the muscles and glands are carried on the efferent nerves.

The autonomic nervous system (ANS)

The autonomic nervous system, has two branches, the sympathetic nervous system (SNS) and the parasympathetic nervous system (PNS). The sympathetic nervous system originates from the thoracic and lumbar regions of the spinal cord and is half of the duo which regulates the ongoing functioning of the body, providing the energy and focus to accomplish necessary internal maintenance and execute life tasks. It also initiates fight and flight responses when the body feels, or is, threatened. The parasympathetic nervous system, which is the other part of the duo, communicates with the body through the vagus nerve, which originates in the brain stem. Its major function is to facilitate the digestion of food and the repair of the body. It is also primarily responsible for the various mechanisms which shut down body functions when the body experiences an inescapable threat, or is primed to feel like it does.

In a healthy, regulated system, the sympathetic and parasympathetic nervous systems balance each other, producing a rhythmic flow from rest to activity. This pattern is illustrated in Figure 1.2, the "window of tolerance" (WOT).

The window of tolerance is the space between the two horizontal lines, where the individual generally feels safe and connected to their body and the external environment. The sympathetic nervous system activation peaks at the top of the curve, indicating maximum energy for activity, and the parasympathetic nervous system is its most activated at the bottom, demonstrating its maximum potential for rest and repair. The regular amplitude is a sign of a regulated autonomic nervous system, where both branches are operating optimally.

This rhythm manifests in at least two important physiological functions: the space between the heartbeats, and the inhalation and exhalation. The heartbeat quickens when the sympathetic nervous system is dominant and slows when the parasympathetic nervous system is dominant. This phenomenon, called heart rate variability (HRV), is a measure of autonomic nervous system health. If it were to be displayed as a graph, a healthy heart rate would look something like the wave. Similarly, in a healthy breathing pattern, the sympathetic nervous system is most activated at the top of the inhale, and the parasympathetic nervous system, at the bottom of the exhale. The term for this is "normal sinus arrhythmia" (Soos & McComb, 2020). In one full breath, the entire range of autonomic activity can be experienced. This autonomic function can be automatic, or intentionally applied, giving the individual some power in influencing their subconscious processes (Shields, 2009).

When an individual senses threat, and its protective resources are not sufficient to maintain feelings of safety, the sympathetic nervous system initiates physiological changes which improve its chances for survival. The major symptoms include:

- Sugar and fat enter the bloodstream, increasing available fuel.

- The respiration rate increases, raising the level of oxygen in the bloodstream.

- Heart rate and blood pressure increase, speeding the delivery of oxygen and fuel to the cells.

- Blood-clotting mechanisms activate, preventing excessive blood loss.

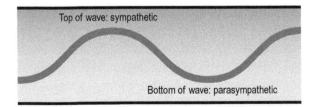

Figure 1.2 Window of tolerance.

- Muscle tone increases, anticipating muscular effort.

- Perspiration increases, in order to regulate the body's temperature.

- The pituitary increases hormonal output to maximize focus.

- The pupils of the eye dilate, offering the widest field of view.

- Short-term attention and alertness increase (Robin, 2009, p. 174).

- Blood is directed to the extremities, rather than to the organs and the brain, to allow for a fight or a flight. This shift puts a hold on digestion, and begins to shut down the higher cognitive functions, which require oxygen and glucose to function (Robin, 2009, p. 17).

During parasympathetic nervous system activation, the reactions are the opposite: saliva flows; the bronchial tubes constrict; digestion accelerates: and the kidneys release urine. More blood is available to fuel brain functioning. In a threatening situation, where escape is impossible, the autonomic nervous system may shift into states of freeze, tonic immobility, or collapsed immobility. In the freeze state, the muscles become rigid, there is a loss of connection with body sensation, an inability to think, difficulty moving the limbs, and some dissociation of the senses from connection with the external world. In the states of immobility, the body goes limp, and the basic physiological processes are slowed to the point where the individual may faint (Kozlowska et al., 2015). These states are tied to the functioning of the dorsal branch of the vagus nerve, discussed later in this chapter and in Chapter 4.

ANS functioning in an acute traumatic situation

Figure 1.3 shows the autonomic nervous system pattern evoked in a crisis, as well as in chronic traumatic disorders. The areas above and below the horizontal line show the jagged pattern of a dysregulated nervous system, extending outside of the window of tolerance. If the individual has a healthy autonomic nervous system, these extremes soon level off and normal oscillation is restored (shown as the curving line within the window). In the unhealed trauma survivor, however, the unbalanced pattern becomes chronic (Sherin & Nemeroff, 2011) and is associated with post-traumatic stress disorder, as well as various mental disorders. In this model, the anxiety disorders, correlated with a high level of sympathetic nervous system arousal, form a spectrum above

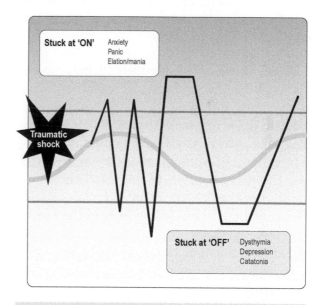

Figure 1.3 Nervous system dysregulation due to traumatic stress.

the window from mild anxiety to mania. The depressive disorders, ranging from dysthymia to catatonia, fall below the window. Anxiety and depressive disorders are often comorbid, a pattern which also appears in this diagram. This condition can occur when the body becomes exhausted when maintaining a high level of sympathetic nervous system arousal, precipitating a crash in its energy level, which manifests as depression.

As an example of the way the autonomic nervous system influences our behavior, let us suppose a well-regulated person is flying to an important business meeting. They breeze through airport security, and then suddenly realize they forgot their coat at the checkpoint. Their sympathetic nervous system will most likely become slightly activated, causing a minor elevation of the heart rate, body temperature, and muscle tension. In this mildly stressed state, this person would likely be open to an offer of help from a kindly airport worker, which would reinforce feelings of safety.

If they are also late for their flight, and are no longer feeling safe, their autonomic nervous system may shift into fight mode, and they are ready to yell at anyone who gets in their way! As they take a deep breath and activate the parasympathetic nervous system, the vagus nerve and the muscles begin to relax, and the autonomic nervous system soon reregulates itself. The neocortex, the thinking part of the brain, can then go back online with a reasonable response and action plan, saying, "I have time to go back and get my coat. It's OK; I won't miss my plane."

However, suppose that in a different scenario at the airport, a person with a chronically dysregulated autonomic nervous system is running late, on their way to the same meeting. They have not adequately prepared for the meeting, and are already feeling stressed, in a low level of the fight-or-flight response. They then forget their coat at the checkpoint and imagine they will have to go through security again. Their dysregulation increases, their breath becomes shallower, and their mind generates images of missing their plane. Even though they know what time it is, they look up at a clock and, for a moment, the hands appear to be one hour later than they actually are. They panic, which increases their dysregulation.

As they become more dysregulated, they begin to perspire, have difficulty thinking, and feel dread. In spite of finally arriving at the gate in time, their autonomic nervous system remains in a state of high alert, imagining the ways that the flight could be delayed or cancelled. This discomfort lessens when they sit down in the plane, but is still present.

The way that brain structures interact explains some of these reactions (Cozolino, 2010, p. 8). For example, when glancing at the clock, this traveler may know what time it is, but remain stuck in a pattern of fight-or-flight reactivity which perpetuates itself, even when there is no real cause (Cozolino, 2010). This individual can immediately trigger themselves by the thought of having to go through security again. In this survival-based reaction, the sympathetic nervous system is primed to fight or flee, based on the individual's imagination, before the information has been processed by the neocortex. That structure evaluates the danger, rather than reacting. An individual in that state may not be able to think clearly, or calm down, for a significant period of time.

Nervous system-informed, trauma-sensitive yoga (NITYA), as well as other approaches to somatic healing, begins with the premise that if an individual can learn to modulate their autonomic nervous system overarousal, bringing it back into the window of tolerance, the symptoms of trauma will diminish. This would leave the client more able to be present and receptive, and to benefit from other, focused trauma treatments (Winblad et al., 2018). Using an example from NITYA, a therapeutic yoga posture may modulate arousal by reducing two related symptoms of PTSD, muscle tension and anxiety, as a result of stretching the muscles, being aware of the breath (Conrad & Roth, 2007). Eventually, an individual may be able to maintain a lower level of muscle tension while tolerating unpleasant sensations.

As I have mentioned, this ability to modulate the ANS is exactly where classical yoga practices, including postures, breathing practices, and relaxation, excel. By using the techniques outlined in this book, the therapist can assist the client in reestablishing a sustained balance between the SNS and PNS, paving the way for recovery from psychological trauma and its accompanying symptoms.

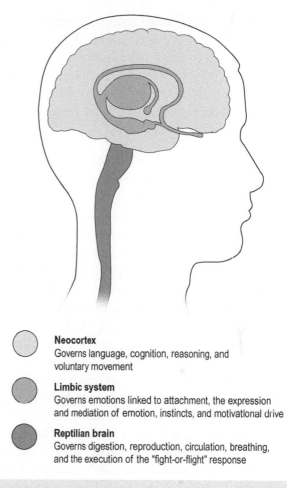

Neocortex
Governs language, cognition, reasoning, and voluntary movement

Limbic system
Governs emotions linked to attachment, the expression and mediation of emotion, instincts, and motivational drive

Reptilian brain
Governs digestion, reproduction, circulation, breathing, and the execution of the "fight-or-flight" response

Figure 1.4 Triune brain model.

The triune brain and trauma processing: background information

In the 1970s, the neuroscientist Paul MacLean presented a model of the brain which he called "the triune brain" (Figure 1.4) (Holden, 1979). While this model is simplistic, it can be used to explain the basic physiology of the brain in simple language. The three parts of the brain which MacLean describes are: the "neocortex," governing language, cognition, reasoning, and voluntary movement; the "limbic brain," which governs emotional reactions, among other functions; and the brain stem, also called the "reptilian brain," which governs the autonomic nervous system and the automatic functions of the body, such as digestion, reproduction, circulation, breathing, and the fight/flight/freeze mechanism (Stangor & Walinga, 2014).

A harmonious relationship between these different parts of the brain allows the individual to be alert, aware, and relaxed at the same time, "moving fluidly between instinct, emotion and rational thought" (Levine, 1997, p. 265). In my view, this is the state that the classic yoga tradition fosters.

Treatment focused on interventions that regulate the primitive brain is classified as a "bottom-up" approach. This approach is in contrast to traditional talk-based psychotherapy, a "top-down" approach, which primarily engages the neocortex, with its executive functions: attention, working memory, planning, reasoning, controlling motivational drives, executive monitoring, reappraising, and meta-awareness (Gard et al., 2014). Neither approach alone can heal the organism; optimal health can be maintained if both approaches work together harmoniously. They can create "conscious evolution," where the emerging somatic material powers the transformation, while the intellect maintains its oversight over the process. (NOTE: The term "conscious evolution" was introduced to me in the Psychosynthesis Counselor Training Program, the Synthesis Center, Amherst, MA, 1986.)

A bottom-up approach uses information from body sensations and emotions to inform decisions and generate behavior, which may be the best intervention, initially, for most trauma survivors. As evidence, brain scans have shown that during a trauma-generated flashback, Broca's area, a part of the brain important for speech production and comprehension, as well as predicting the consequences of one's actions, shuts down to some degree. This means that the individual may not be able to speak about a traumatic memory, or use the experience to inform future decisions, until they have processed the experience on the somatic level (van der Kolk, 2014, p. 43; Cozolino, 2010, p. 6). The processing can proceed when the client becomes more aware of body sensations (Tsur et al., 2018.) Research on the effect of trauma on the brain, as well as the work of Dr. Stephen Porges on polyvagal theory, described later in this chapter, further illuminate why bottom-up processing is crucial to autonomic nervous system health.

One of yoga's strengths is that it functions as both a top-down and a bottom-up approach. As the NITYA practitioner sends instructions from the neocortex to the body to move in a particular way, top-down processing is strengthened. In contrast, by feeling the sensations generated in a yoga pose, the client can further develop bottom-up awareness, termed "interoception." The heightened awareness of sensations can engage the neocortex, which strengthens the connection between top-down and bottom-up processes.

The importance of interoception in trauma healing and in NITYA

The importance of interoception, the observation of inner processes, was originally recognized by neuroscientist Antonio Damasio, who developed the "somatic marker hypothesis," which postulates that rational thinking is partially based on the experience of body sensations and emotions, which serve as a major source of the data on which a decision rests (Damasio, 2005). Interoception is a key to self-care, alerting an individual to their bodily needs. For example, the trauma survivor may work to exhaustion, disconnected from the signals that the body is sending that it needs rest. This behavior can result in illness. (NOTE: The areas of the brain that are devoted to self-awareness (the medial prefrontal cortex) and body awareness (the insula) often have shrunk in people with chronic post-traumatic stress disorder (van der Kolk, foreword to Levine, 2015, p. xv).)

The connection with sensations is an essential part of identifying emotional states. For example, someone who feels sad may experience tightness in the chest, a heaviness behind the eyes, a lump in the throat. By focusing on experiencing emotion through sensation, the emotion may be easier to describe, its impact can be less overwhelming, and the individual can remain more present while feeling it.

Recovery can begin when the client learns to use interoception to become aware of the body's current state. On a deeper level, they can recognize and interrupt "somatic loops," which are composed of sensations, thoughts, memories, and actions related to unprocessed traumatic memories (Poppa & Bechara, 2018). Each component of the loop influences the others ("How do you feel? Lecture by Bud Craig," 2009). For example, changes in the degree of muscle tension influence thoughts and feelings. The skillful use of interoception can eventually change the way survivors experience their life. Developing this ability highlights the importance of a bottom-up, mind/body practice like yoga.

Dr. Stephen Porges and polyvagal theory in healing trauma

Dr. Stephen Porges has proposed a physiological model, polyvagal theory (PVT), which gives insight into the body's survival mechanisms. It is based on the functioning of the vagus nerve, which is the most influential of the cranial nerves, and has received the most attention in trauma therapy (Schwartz, 2019).

The vagus nerve, the 10th cranial nerve, is the main pathway of the parasympathetic nervous system, and the longest nerve in the body (Figure 1.5). It emerges from the brain stem and connects with the body's major vital organs. Approximately 80% of the vagus nerve fibers are afferent, meaning that they transmit information from the body to the brain, a bottom-up function.

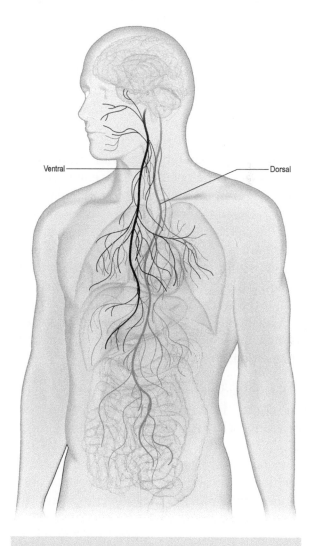

Figure 1.5 The vagus nerve.

The brain can interpret the message, then relay it back through the nerve, influencing behavior.

While the vagus is often described as a single nerve, it is actually a pair, consisting of the ventral (front) vagal complex (VVC) and the dorsal (back) vagal complex (DVC), each with different pathways through the body. The ventral vagal complex regulates the muscles above the diaphragm, which connect to the facial features, soft palate, pharynx, larynx, middle ear, esophagus, heart and lungs – all features which are active when we are socially engaged with another human being (Dykema, 2006). The dorsal branch connects to the organs below the diaphragm which primarily control digestion.

Social engagement is possible when the individual feels safe in their body and their environment. Physiologically, in the state of social engagement the ventral vagal complex is predominant and the sympathetic/parasympathetic nervous system arousal is balanced and regulated, functioning within the window of tolerance. In that scenario, the sympathetic nervous system can provide the necessary energy and focus to accomplish life tasks, and the parasympathetic nervous system can facilitate healthy digestion, rest, and rejuvenation.

The individual, who is said to be in "ventral vagus," is calm, able to self-soothe, has relaxed muscles, and can distinguish the human voice from other background sounds. They characteristically have relaxed facial muscles, a soothing voice, and a variable heart rate. These features subliminally communicate safety to other nervous systems.

Porges termed the nervous system's tendency to assess for danger "neuroception." Neuroception is an unconscious neural process, distinct from perception, which can distinguish safety or danger in the environment (Porges, 2011). If an environment triggers feelings of unsafety, the organism activates its sympathetic nervous system, with its fight-or-flight impulse. When fighting or fleeing is impossible, the dorsal vagal complex initiates the last line of defense, an "immobilization response," where the prefrontal cortex goes offline, and there is a shutdown of emotions, sensations, and biological processes (Levine, 2015, p. 55). (NOTE: In this model, the shutdown is seen as a causative factor in mental disorders such as post-traumatic stress disorder, depression, and bulimia nervosa (Gillig & Sanders, 2010; Blechert et al., 2007).)

The role of the cranial nerves in social engagement

Five of the 12 cranial nerves (numbers 3, 5, 7, 9, and 11) work in conjunction with the vagus nerve (#10) to create the physiological basis for social engagement (Porges, 2009). These nerves support the PNS by controlling the movement, and degree of tension, of specific muscles and transmitting sensory information to the brain. Interestingly, many yogic interventions work in conjunction with the cranial nerves. They will be identified in Chapters 3 and 4.

Cranial nerve #3, the oculomotor nerve, regulates eye movement, one aspect of interpersonal connection. It also governs the oculocardiac reflex, which decreases the pulse rate in the circulatory system when the eyeball is gently compressed, through its connection with the vagus nerve (Robin, 2009, p. 192).

Two nerves, the trigeminal nerve (or cranial nerve #5) and facial nerve #7, influence the degree of tension or relaxation in the face and mouth, an important indicator of sympathetic/parasympathetic nervous system balance. Relaxing the jaw can increase parasympathetic nervous system tone and send a reassuring message of safety to anyone interacting with that individual (Robin, 2009).

The glossopharyngeal nerve, cranial nerve #9, receives sensory information from parts of the tongue, carotids, tonsils, and middle ear, and innervates parasympathetic nervous system fibers which aid in digestion and rest. Relaxing the tongue can increase parasympathetic nervous system tone and communicate safety to others (Robin, 2009). Because of its connection with the middle ear, this nerve helps to distinguish the sound of the human voice from background noises, which can influence a person's perceived safety level. It also registers danger when hearing certain low-register sounds (Howes, 2013).

Cranial nerve #11 is responsible for controlling the muscles which turn the head, a component of human communication. The state of this nerve is another determinate of the degree of safety which an individual communicates to others and experiences for themselves (Porges, 2009, p. 588). (NOTE: Parasympathetic nervous system-related nerves also emanate from the sacral plexus, located from the second to fourth sacral segments (S2–S4), which regulate sexual function, urination, and bowel movements. This area has not yet received attention in trauma treatment.)

Yoga for self-regulation

Traditionally, self-regulation refers to the processes by which individuals control or direct their thoughts, emotions, and actions to achieve their goals ("Self-Regulation", 2020).

Research has shown that a yoga practice allows the individual to endure more physical stress or intense emotional reactivity before the ANS becomes dysregulated. The ANS can also elicit parasympathetic tone more rapidly in a stressful situation in a yoga practitioner than in someone who does not practice yoga (Gard et al., 2014). These benefits improve the individual's ability to remain calm and present

Other developments in neuroscience which support healing through NITYA

Mirror neurons and interpersonal neurobiology

The importance of the state of an individual's nervous system in facilitating health is underscored by the study of interpersonal neurobiology and of neuroplasticity of the brain.

The field of interpersonal neurobiology partly rests upon the discovery of mirror neurons, a type of brain cell that responds similarly whether we perform an action or witness someone else perform the same action (Winerman, 2005). They were first identified in the early 1990s by the Italian neurophysiologist Dr. Giancomo Rizzolatti and his colleagues at the University of Parma, Italy (Rizzolatti et al., 2006). They found that individual neurons in the brains of macaque monkeys fired both when the monkeys grabbed an object and also when the monkeys watched another primate grab the same object (Winerman, 2005).

When applied to humans, they indicate that a significant number of our interactions are unconscious. We may internalize the gestures, emotional tone, facial expressions, thoughts, and attitudes of others without choosing to or realizing it (Siegel, 2006). These subconscious messages can determine whether others feel safe with us or not.

Neuroplasticity

Recent research has proven the power of our conscious decisions to modify neuronal networks in the brain. This phenomenon is called "neuroplasticity." An example is modifications which occur in the brain when we learn to play the piano. Initially, when the individual starts to play, new neurons are created in the brain to govern the fine movements of the fingers. After regular practice, the individual neurons within the map become more efficient and their connections stronger, so that eventually fewer neurons are required to perform the same task (Doidge, 2007), or as psychologist Donald Hebb theorized, "neurons that fire together, wire together" (Hebb, 2002).

The same principles work in yoga practice, where practitioners are streamlining and amending existing networks, and creating new ones. Practicing yoga regularly, with a focus on the body sensations and breathing pattern, can help to rewire traumatized parts of the brain, and allow more capacity for new perceptions. The yoga tradition itself recognized the relationship between our thoughts and attitudes, and our embodied experience. In the words of Swami Sivananda, "Your body is your objectified thought. When your thoughts change, the body will also change" (Sivananda, 1980). And I would like to add, from my own experience, that when your body changes, your thoughts will also change.

Research also shows that it is easier to establish new neural networks if one is paying close attention to what one does. This is crucial because "the focus of attention enables new synaptic connections to be established … neuroplasticity may be the fundamental way in which psychotherapy alters the brain" (Siegel, 2006, p. 249). One strength of yoga and other meditative traditions is that they train us to pay close attention to what is happening in the present moment.

Negativity bias

Researchers have found that, on the cognitive level, due to the need to ensure our continued survival, highly-charged, negative experiences are given priority in memory storage, producing a "negativity bias" (Vaish et al., 2008). Cognitive therapist Aaron Beck identified a similar tendency, postulating that evolution favors an "anxious gene" (Cozolino, 2008). This tendency exacerbates the negative effects of trauma. That is one reason why it is detrimental to focus excessively either on negative experiences from the past or on fantasies about the future, which strengthen their connection and influence in the neural network, rather than on creating positive connections in the present (Doidge, 2007, p. 47).

To overcome this tendency, the therapist can help the client to shift away from a focus on negative experience, and toward an inner resource. The best ways to do that differ from person to person. They might include assuming a yoga pose which is regulating, focusing on the rhythm of the breath, experiencing the caring quality of the voice of the therapist/teacher, or remembering a positive moment from the past.

Every positive experience can become a resource for healing.

A client can experiment with this strategy by listing as many positive experiences as he/she can recall. When, at some point, the client's thoughts shift to an incident that is unhealed, he or she can stay there for a moment and then consciously shift back to a positive experience to avoid retraumatization. I have found that, over time, the more often the positive states are experienced, the more resilient a person can become, and the easier it is to maintain them. Psychologist Rick Hanson refers to this approach as "installing the good" (Hanson, 2014).

The NITYA healing model

The NITYA healing model is summarized in Figure 1.1, presented at the beginning of this chapter. It was originally inspired by Dan Siegel's concept of "the window of tolerance" (Siegel, 1999). The word "yoga" itself means "union," and the charts which follow (Figures 1.6–1.9) illustrate the union of somatic, emotional, mental, and energetic dimensions of human experience, from a polarized, dysregulated state to a unified, centered state. To emphasize the power of yoga, I have changed the name of the regulated section of the window of tolerance to the "yoga zone."

NITYA, accompanied by some form of supportive psychotherapy or yoga therapy, is designed to heal these dysregulations, bringing them into the "yoga zone," so that the individual can live in harmony with him or herself. This approach can also widen the yoga zone, so that experiences which were once deregulating, no longer are.

Looking at the chart

The NITYA healing model offers the therapist a map of the client's level of functioning in different areas, and a visual tool which can guide treatment planning (Figures 1.6–1.9). This model highlights the interdependence of the physical, emotional, cognitive, and energetic levels, which operate together (Sullivan et al., 2018). It offers an overview of the effects of polarization, and the potential for healing. On the physical level, the polarities are sympathetic nervous system overarousal at one extreme, and parasympathetic nervous system dorsal-vagal shutdown at the other. On the emotional level, anxiety-related emotions, including panic and rage, are present in the overarousal zone, and depression-related symptoms, such as shame and guilt, appear in the underarousal zone. On the cognitive level, various cognitive distortions operate in both polarities. In the energetic realm, the imbalances are presented in the language of the gunas, described in the Vedas as the qualities of all matter. Rajasic energy has similar qualities to sympathetic nervous system overactivation; tamasic energy is equivalent to dorsal-vagal shutdown.

The resolution of the polarities occurs in the yoga zone. On the physical level, it manifests as nervous system regulation, where the sympathetic nervous system and parasympathetic nervous system arousal are balanced and oscillating. Emotionally, it is characterized as contentment, the result of knowing that we can experience difficult emotions and move

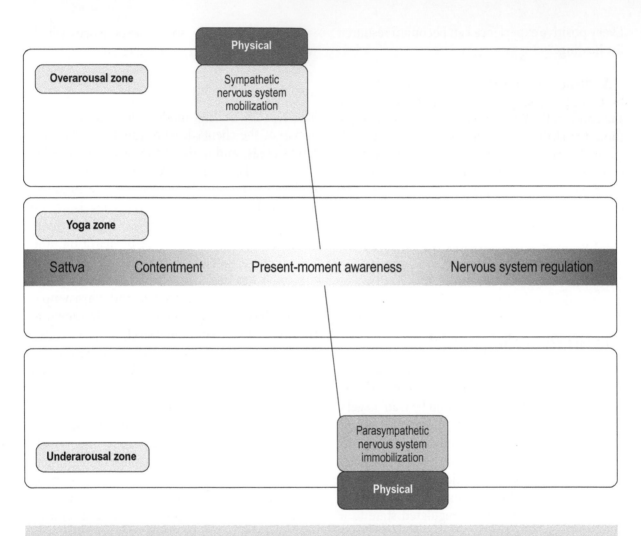

Figure 1.6 NITYA Healing Model, Physical Polarity. On the physical level, the polarities are: sympathetic nervous system overarousal at one extreme and parasympathetic dorsal-vagal shutdown at the other. The healing synthesis, represented in the yoga zone, is nervous system regulation.

Physical polarity

For most clients, I recommend the physical level as the major therapeutic focus. This modality includes the yogic postures, breathing practices, the initial stages of the yogic sleep. These interventions were designed to regulate the autonomic nervous system, and are much easier to work with, and more powerful than, a suggestion to change one's feeling state, or mental state. When done with concentration, the physiological interventions can naturally calm emotions and quiet thoughts. Then deeper neuroception, and self-connection, is possible. This shift can pave the way for trauma healing.

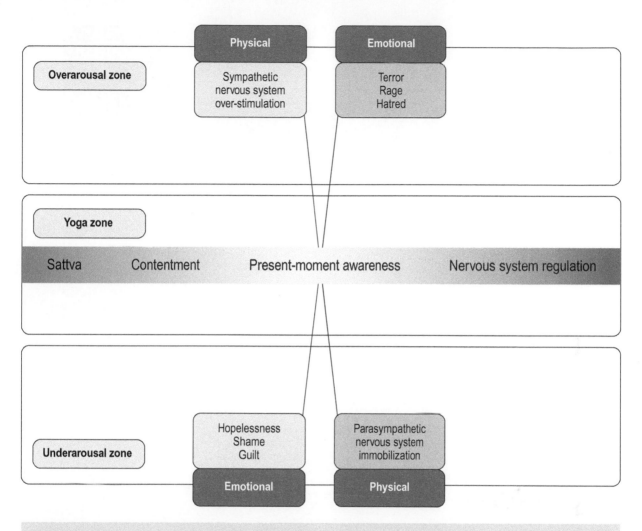

Figure 1.7 NITYA Healing Model, Emotional Polarity. On the emotional level, anxiety-related symptoms, including panic, are present in the overarousal zone, with corresponding emotions such as fear, terror, and rage. The depression-related symptoms, with the corresponding emotions of hopelessness, shame, and guilt, appear in the underarousal area. When these polarities are healed, the result is contentment, included in the yoga zone.

Emotional polarity

In many individuals, emotions are strong and constantly changing. With these changes come frequent autonomic shifts which influence muscle tension, hormone and neurotransmitter levels, thoughts, and attitudes, to name a few, and can have a negative impact on health. The individual may look outside of him or herself, to substances and/or relationships, for stability. When the autonomic nervous system is regulated, the emotions begin to calm. As time goes on, the individual may notice an inner stability, a more secure platform from which to act. They can experience the world more objectively, being aware of more options. Then the emotions become guides, rather than masters, and contentment can grow.

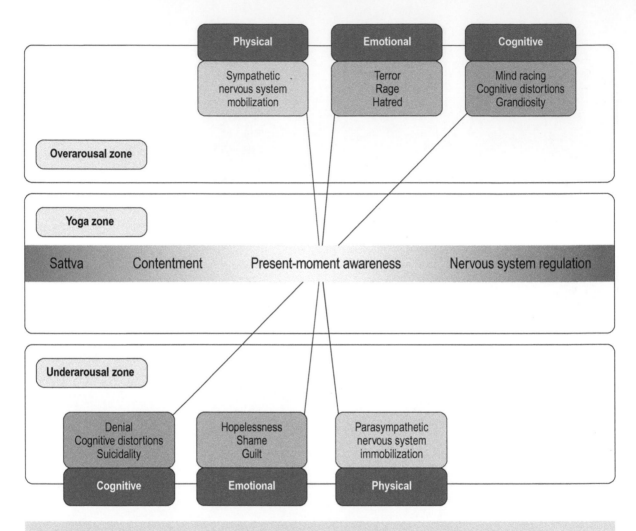

Figure 1.8 NITYA Healing Model, Cognitive Polarity. On the cognitive level, various cognitive distortions operate in both polarities. I describe the healing as present-moment awareness.

Mental polarity

Life can become hellish when the mind is overactive and the thoughts keep racing on. They drag emotions along with them, possibly increasing feelings of isolation, desperation, and fatigue. Thoughts may drift to illusions of grandiosity or, at the other extreme, suicidality. Physiological symptoms such as insomnia and irritability may manifest. When the autonomic nervous system is regulated, life can be experienced moment-to-moment, with each moment offering new possibilities, and opening more potential for present-moment awareness.

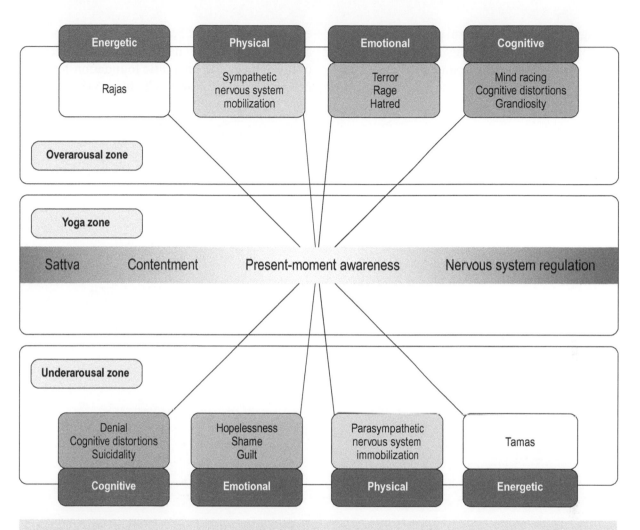

Figure 1.9 The NITYA Healing Model, Energetic Polarity.
Energetic polarity
While the gunas do not fit well into the mind/body/spirit categories, I am conceptualizing them as operating in the energetic realm. One of their functions is to coordinate the activity of the autonomic nervous system states, when impacted by the practices contained in the limbs of Raja Yoga (Sullivan et al., 2018).

through them, rather than getting stuck. On the cognitive level, healing manifests as present-moment awareness, a state where the mind is energized and peaceful. The resolution of the energetic polarity is Sattva, the guna of peace and harmony. The next chapter provides a philosophical and energetic foundation for the practices which follow in Chapters 3 through 5.

Raja Yoga and yogic subtle anatomy as a foundation for NITYA therapeutic yoga

The NITYA approach to Raja Yoga

As I studied the confluence of classical yoga, somatic experiencing, and neurobiological research, I was astonished at the congruences that emerged. This chapter lays a foundation for a discussion of those similarities, with presentations on the royal path of yoga, Raja Yoga, followed by the subtle physiology of the autonomic nervous system (ANS), and relevant studies from the field of neuroscience.

Raja Yoga with an ANS twist

Raja Yoga, the "royal path," is described in the Yoga Sutras of Patanjali, a set of 196 aphorisms or "sutras," believed to have been communicated through oral traditions and codified in approximately 400 BCE. Sutra number two is considered to be the keystone of yoga practice. The many different translations, when distilled, define yoga as the stilling of the mind. This sutra is central to the definition of yoga as a practice primarily intended to bring about the transformation of the mind by calming its agitations. This focus links Raja Yoga and the practices which have developed from it with current medical concerns about the effect of trauma and stress on one's mental health.

The goal of NITYA, which is based on Raja Yoga, is to optimize mental health by applying yogic techniques that regulate the ANS. According to research on state-dependent learning, when the ANS is regulated, the client feels physically and emotionally safe, the neo-cortex is on-line, and optimal learning is possible (Staal, 2004). The client in this state can engage in and optimally

benefit from trauma-focused psychotherapy (Shapiro, 2018; Fenn & Byrne, 2013).

Raja Yoga outlines a path of spiritual development, often depicted as limbs on a tree. Figure 2.1 is one representation of the ascending limbs of Raja Yoga, with their eight levels of practice. It includes a brief description of the limbs of Raja Yoga; further detail about them appears here and in later chapters.

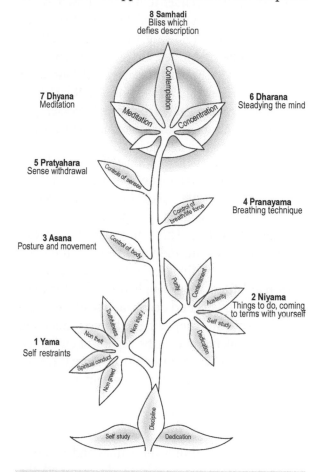

Figure 2.1 Raja Yoga tree.

Chapter 2

Yamas and niyamas

The first two limbs, the yamas and niyamas, are composed of 10 moral and ethical principles. In a contemporary interpretation, the yamas include having reverence toward all living things, so as not to do any harm to oneself or others; being truthful, disciplined in the expenditure of one's energy, and generous. The niyamas (#2), practices for inner spiritual development, prescribe cultivating clarity and authenticity, contentment, self-discipline, self-study, and surrender to a higher power, or, in secular terms, to the path of the highest good for all living things. Practicing these precepts allows the practitioner to build a life of integrity, which I see as a prerequisite for inner peace. (I have been inspired by Nischala Devi's book *The Secret Path of Yoga*, for breaking new ground in the contemporary interpretation of these foundational practices.)

The focus on virtues in these first two limbs may seem tangential to current trends in yoga or in modern life. However, when viewed from a neurobiological perspective, they have considerable value. The cultivation of positive qualities can help an individual build self-esteem and maximize feelings of wellbeing, increasing ANS regulation. When applied to life situations, they can facilitate good decision making and connection to others. They can also form a foundation for "moral safety," one of the aspects of embodied safety, which develops in a culture where there is a consensus as to what constitutes right and wrong (Shea, M.J., Biodynamic Perceptions of Safety, on-line course, 1/18/21).

Conversely, devaluing the yamas and niyamas can lead to some degree of inner dis-ease, with the accompanying ANS dysregulation. At the same time, however, as with all techniques, working with the yamas and niyamas may not suit everyone, and may even increase feelings of shame and guilt in some clients. Because of this, they need to be applied sensitively.

The next two limbs, asana and pranayama, are the practices that are the most engaged with the body.

Asana

Limb #3 is asana, the Sanskrit word for "steady and comfortable pose." Asana was originally intended as a preparation for meditation, helping to maintain a healthy body and a focused mind, which are the prerequisites for this practice (Satchidananda, 1970, p. xix). NITYA uses yoga postures not as training for meditation practice, although that may be a side benefit, but to help a trauma survivor heal. They do this through their ability to energize and/or relax the practitioner, based on what the ANS needs to regulate itself. This is accomplished through the skillful use of moderately-paced motor movement, which upregulates the SNS, and a focus on slow, deep breaths and muscle releasing postures, which downregulate the PNS. The postures can also help the client to more deeply feel their body sensations (called interoception), which increases the sense of self; know where they are in space (proprioception); sense if they are safe or not (neuroception), and take effective action to maintain their safety. In Chapter 3, you will find guidelines on choosing the most effective posture to achieve the desired state.

Pranayama (breath control)

Limb #4, "prânâyâma," is concerned with the control of life energy. *Prana* is the Sanskrit word for "life energy," and *yama* means "control." Such control is achieved through a variety of breathing techniques that direct the movement of prana through the body. In the NITYA system, the goal of pranayama practice is to regulate the subtle and gross nervous systems, explained in more detail in this chapter. Chapter 4, presents specific breathing practices that facilitate this balance.

Pratyahara

The next limb, #5, "pratyâhâra," which means "sense withdrawal," is a withdrawal of one's focus and energy from the external world to the internal one. For the spiritual aspirant, yoga nidra offers a doorway to higher states of consciousness, and an opportunity to dismantle a culturally constructed personality. The NITYA system adapts this practice for trauma survivors by offering practices which deepen their experience of embodiment, while gradually connecting more deeply with inner states. This practice is presented in more detail in Chapter 7.

In my trauma-sensitive work, in general, I emphasize practices from limbs three through five which increase the experience of embodiment. For most trauma survivors, it is these practices which are most beneficial, at least initially, because they offer the practitioner an increased opportunity to experience their sensations, as well as grounding and connection with the external environment. Once survivors have made a solid connection with their body sensations, and have established stable resources in their life, they may benefit from more subtle practices.

Dharana

I consider a regulated ANS to be a prerequisite for the three limbs which follow pratyahara: dharana, dhyana, and samadhi. The first of these, dharana, limb #6, is best described as "concentration."

It involves being able to direct the mind to willfully focus on present-moment experience, concentrating its energy the way a magnifying glass concentrates the sun's energy (Satchidananda, 1970, p. xxvii). An example of this practice is staring at a candle flame. It can therefore be counterproductive for the individual with a dysregulated ANS, as it can magnify the dysregulation.

Dhyana and samadhi

Once the yoga student has established an ability to concentrate, he or she can practice limb #7, called "dhyana," or "meditation," which is focused on developing the mind's ability to expand beyond discursive thought and rest in the space between the thoughts. Another way to describe that ability is the cultivation of the habit of increasing the time lag between the thought or sensation, and the internal response to it. With a more regulated response, there is an increased steadiness of mind and less ANS overactivation. The ultimate goal of meditation in the Yoga Sutras is samâdhi, a sustained state of pure awareness.

Each of the limbs of Raja Yoga is both a building block to the next, and a complete practice in itself. For example, if a student or client is performing a yoga posture with full concentration and awareness of the breath, undisturbed by discursive thoughts, then he or she is gaining the benefits of practicing asana, pranayama, and meditation simultaneously.

In the spirit of ahimsa, or non-injury, the first tenet of the yamas, I want to emphasize the importance of the therapist learning yogic interventions from a well-trained teacher, and then having their own practice. If teaching, the therapist should teach the practices with attention to accuracy and simple wording, while observing the client's responses. Anyone interested in using the NITYA model might consider taking additional trainings to supplement this text in order to use this model more flexibly in a clinical setting, including taking a yoga teacher's training program.

These foundational practices are capped by beliefs which I consider to be the bedrock of yoga philosophy: that the human being is inherently good, and this goodness, even when hidden beneath layers of ignorance, can be retrieved; that the body is intelligent and self-regulating; that inner blocks and disharmonies can be overcome; and finally, that each person is an important part of a greater whole.

Yoga as energy psychology

Yoga, seen in a different framework, is a complete system of energy psychology. As discussed above, yogic texts describe a subtle energy, prana, which interpenetrates our physical body. Classic yoga focuses on the management of prana, which determines the state of health of the organism. By becoming more attentive to it – and enhancing and directing its flow through yoga practices – practitioners and clients can invigorate the body and mind, develop an expanded inner awareness, and become open to the possibility of reaching deeper states of healing (Anderson, 2013).

In this model, prana travels through seven ascending subtle energy centers called "chakras" or wheels. Each one is located at the convergence points of many energy currents in the body and in proximity to the seven major glands of the physical body (although there is no scientific evidence that the chakras and glands are connected). The chakras are also associated with the resolution of psychological milestones which can be compared to Maslow's Hierarchy of Needs, from the most basic to the transcendent.

The state of the first chakra, "muladhara" (meaning "root support"), is said to determine trust vs. mistrust; the second, "svadhistana" (meaning "self-sustaining"), governs sexuality and creativity vs. inhibition. The third, "manipura" (meaning "full of gems"), determines personal power vs. disempowerment. The fourth, "anahata" (meaning "that which cannot be destroyed"), illuminates the polarities of compassion vs. criticism. The fifth, "vishuddha" (meaning "extraordinarily pure"), deals with self-expression vs. fear. The sixth, "ajna" (meaning "command"), beyond polarities, governs intellectual discrimination. The seventh, "sahasrara" (meaning "1,000 spokes"), guides transcendence.

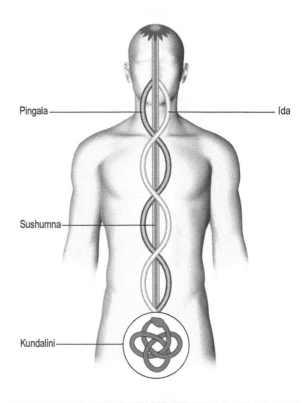

Figure 2.2 Major subtle nerve channels.

According to the Upanishads, a network of 72,000 subtle nerves, called nadis, interpenetrate the physical body, and converge at the chakras (Figure 2.2). Two of the major nadis emerge from the base of the spine and cross at each chakra. One of them, the "ida," meaning "comfort" in Sanskrit, ends at the left nostril; the other, the "pingala", meaning "golden" or "solar," ends at the right. A third, central channel, called the "sushumna," meaning "very gracious" or "kind," located near the spine, travels straight up the subtle body to the top of the head. There is speculation that the ida and pingala nadis are subtle manifestations of the sympathetic and parasympathetic nervous systems (Mishra, 1959, p. 85; Iyengar, 1988, p. 132).

These major nadis emerge from the kundalini, a storehouse of spiritual energy located at the base of the spine. The Shakti and Tantric traditions of Hinduism teach that when the kundalini is activated, this potent energy travels up the sushumna, opening the chakras and transforming consciousness as it goes (Saraswati & Hiti, 1984, pp. 34–36; Radha, 1978).

The awakening of the kundalini can be an organic process, the outcome of years of yoga practice and subtle nerve refinement, which gradually expands a person's awareness. It can also be activated suddenly, before a person's gross and subtle nervous systems are ready, which can then create symptoms of mental illness. This condition was labeled as a "spiritual emergency" by psychiatrist Stanislav Grof and his wife Christina, when differentiating it from a psychotic break, which can manifest similar symptoms (Grof & Grof, 1992).

A traumatic experience can activate the kundalini, blasting someone onto a "spiritual path" (Grof & Grof, 1992; Sannella, 1987). This sudden activation can create imbalances on the physical, emotional, and energetic levels. If handled sensitively and supportively, in conjunction with psychotherapy and, perhaps, a consultation with a practitioner of Ayurveda or Chinese medicine, this type of experience can lead to "post-traumatic growth," which can open the doorway to greater integration of the personality. If handled badly, though, it can lead to further disintegration.

The gunas

The gunas are defined as the three basic qualities of nature. They are an important component of Indian philosophy, as well as a possible correlative to the Western understanding of the functioning of the autonomic nervous system. The Bhagavad Gita, a major Hindu scripture, offers a description of the gunas, categorized as rajas (mobilizing), tamas (stabilizing) and sattva (sustaining) (Easwaran, 2007, pp. 43–47). When in balance, the gunas operate in harmony. When they are unbalanced, and an individual is in an excessively rajasic state, the body is agitated, and the mind can be angry, fearful, demanding, and impatient. In an excessively tamasic state, the body is sluggish and the mind is dull, negatively oriented, and inflexible. Sattva is the desired state, expressing purity, flexibility, and peace. One goal of a yogic lifestyle is to transform excessive tamas into rajas and, then, when enough energy has been built to fuel transformation, from rajas into sattva (Khemka et al., 2011; Zimmer & Campbell, 1990). This transformation can be supported by cultivating regular living habits; spending time in nature; eating a vegetarian diet; living in a peaceful, clean environment; choosing wholesome entertainment; and, as much as possible, associating with well-regulated people.

Qualitatively, the gunas can be interpreted to correspond to ANS states. In a groundbreaking research paper, *Yoga Therapy and Polyvagal Theory: The Convergence of Traditional Wisdom and Contemporary Neuroscience for Self-Regulation and Resilience*, yoga therapists, in collaboration with neuroscientist Stephen Porges, originator of polyvagal theory, describe the gunas in these terms (Sullivan et al., 2018). The gunas comprise

the fourth polarity of the NITYA Healing Model. A hyper-vigilant, sympathetic-dominant state, located above the "yoga zone" on the NITYA Healing Model chart, could be correlated with a rajasic state. The area of the chart associated with dorsal vagal shutdown, represented below the "yoga zone," could be seen as a tamasic state. The yoga zone in the middle, with a smooth oscillation between the SNS and PNS activation,

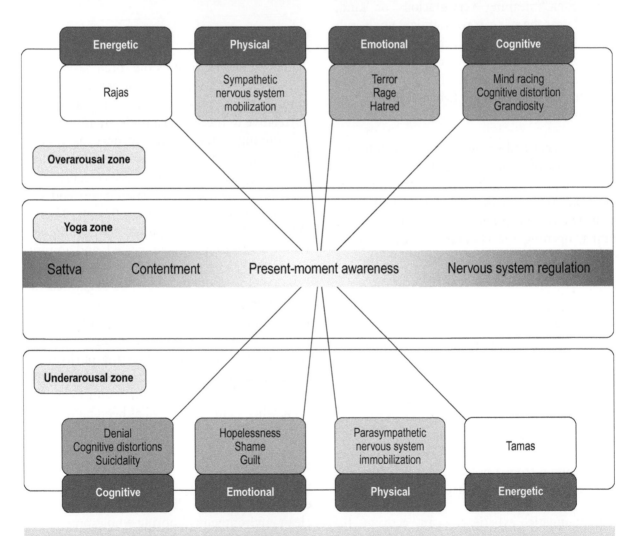

Figure 2.3 NITYA healing model, energetic polarity.

could be seen as a sattvic state which maximizes a health-affirming connection within oneself, and between oneself and others (Sullivan et al., 2018).

An explanation of the chart is now complete.

The difference between yoga for spiritual development and therapeutic yoga

Because yoga has the power to dysregulate as well as regulate the ANS, I feel it is important to distinguish the goal of classical yoga, which is, in my opinion, spiritual transformation, from the goal of NITYA, which is the gradual regulation of the autonomic nervous system.

On the physical level, spiritual transformation begins by using physical/energetic practices to catalyze sympathetic arousal, rousing the energy of tamas, and transforming it into rajas. The intensity of such a practice can heat the body and open various blocks to the free flow of energy. According to yoga therapist Gary Kraftsow, "the means and methods of personal practice that we suggest ... are all designed to help us build sufficient energy to break free of our conditioned responses" (Kraftsow, 2002, p. 20).

Examples of stimulating practices include a routine which focuses on continuous movement, primarily performed standing; the "breath of fire," or "breath of joy," with forceful inhales and/or exhales, routinely taught as an energizing breathing practice; the common practice of breath retention, which may be an invitation for the kundalini to rise; and the practice of bandhas, or "energy locks," which are designed to concentrate

energy (the latter two to be discussed further in Chapter 4). When taught to a regulated person, the individual can feel calmed and energized after this type of practice. However, overstimulation of the SNS, producing or increasing symptoms of dysregulation, can result when these techniques are practiced by individuals in the process of healing from trauma, or who simply have highly sensitive nervous systems.

In my opinion, the lower branches of Raja Yoga, skillfully applied, have the potential to balance and heal the wounds of traumatized individuals, and are therefore therapeutic. The higher branches of the yogic system, limbs #6–#8, can transcend the focus on embodiment for ANS regulation, the theories of polyvagal theory, and the domain of social engagement, and reach for a level of intrapersonal subtlety which has not yet been explored, or researched in depth, in the field of psychology. (It is possible that this frontier may be the domain of the therapeutic use of psychedelic drugs and other altered states of consciousness, such as Stanislav Grof's Holotropic Breathwork and shamanic journeying.)

For these reasons, I have a strong bias toward recommending grounding, embodied practices for individuals recovering from various levels of trauma, adapted to the capacities of each person. In upcoming chapters, you will see this perspective resonating in the recommendations for working with yoga postures and breathing practices which work with the SNS/PNS balance; in the suggestion of offering yoga nidra in four stages, keyed to the individual's progress; and in the emphasis on teaching embodied versions of meditation.

In our first session, Emily reports that she has had some experiences in yoga classes which set her back in her healing process. She experienced one teacher as authoritarian, ignoring her expression of discomfort while in several poses. In another class, the teacher touched her without asking for her permission, which precipitated a panic attack. In spite of these experiences, Emily believes that yoga can help her to quiet her mood swings and reduce her anxiety, and she is willing to enter a yoga-informed approach to psychotherapy.

This chapter focuses on the basics of nervous system-informed, trauma-sensitive yoga postures (NITYA), which offer the psychotherapist, yoga therapist, or yoga teacher yogic interventions which are based on their influence on the client's autonomic state. (The terms trauma-sensitive and trauma-informed are used interchangeably in this text as their meaning is the same.)

As I mentioned in the vignette above, the importance of trauma sensitivity emerged out of accounts of trauma survivors being retraumatized in yoga classes, where the instructor may have touched them, and moved parts of their body into an uncomfortable position, without permission; instructed them to assume poses that emphasized exposing sexually vulnerable parts of their body; and, in general, encouraged them to override their body wisdom, in favor of complying with the instructions. This approach can rekindle survivors' submission patterns, leaving them feeling helpless. If the teacher is male, it can also reinforce oppressive gender-based roles.

Trauma sensitivity is an important aspect of the teaching of yoga in general, as well as in a specifically therapeutic context, since there is

evidence that a large percentage of yoga students have dealt with trauma in some form. In the Trauma-Informed Lens Yoga Survey, conducted informally in 2016 by the Yoga and Body Image Coalition, 93% of the 132 students sampled had experienced some form of trauma, as measured by the "Life Events Checklist" (Blake et al., 1995; YBIcoalition.com). A study in 2017 replicated these results (YBIcoalition.com). David Emerson and his colleagues at The Trauma Center in Brookline, Massachusetts, recognized this need and developed an approach to meet it which they labelled "Trauma-Sensitive Yoga." NITYA developed out of an early iteration of Trauma-Sensitive Yoga, integrated with the physiology of the ANS.

I consider the greatest contribution of Emerson's trauma-sensitive yoga to NITYA to be in the use of invitational and interoceptive language. Invitational phrases such as "when you are," "if you like," "I invite you," and "would it be alright?" empower the individual to make their own choices. Interoceptive language, such as "how does it feel when," or "what is it like when you," encourage the individual to connect with the internal experience of each pose, which helps them to recognize and articulate their felt experience, on and off the yoga mat (Emerson et al., 2009).

The interoceptive focus in this approach includes awareness of general body sensations, breathing patterns, sensations of energetic flow, emotional states, and cognitions. This approach contrasts with a focus on alignment and precision of execution, which can be important for injury prevention, and for applying yoga to medical conditions, but is not as useful to most people seeking to reconnect with their inner experience. NITYA focuses on this goal, training the client to be aware of their ANS states. It offers them the skills to reset their ANS when activation has gone above or below the window of tolerance, as well as for self-soothing.

Working with NITYA factors in choosing interventions

NITYA offers mental health and yoga professionals guidance on which yogic-based interventions to use at key moments in the session, when the ANS is becoming dysregulated, and how to apply them. After determining that the client has an ANS imbalance, either chronic or acute, and is willing to explore an embodied approach, the therapist can work with the four dimensions of the yoga postures listed below in an interoceptive manner, to create optimal interventions. They include: (1) intention, (2) shape, (3) pace, and (4) effort (Figure 3.1).

1 Setting the intention, which is generally either to lower or raise the SNS or PNS charge, and then to balance the two in order

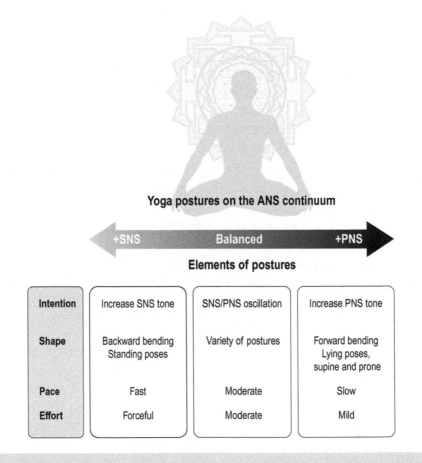

Yoga postures on the ANS continuum

+SNS   Balanced   +PNS

Elements of postures

Intention	Increase SNS tone	SNS/PNS oscillation	Increase PNS tone
Shape	Backward bending Standing poses	Variety of postures	Forward bending Lying poses, supine and prone
Pace	Fast	Moderate	Slow
Effort	Forceful	Moderate	Mild

Figure 3.1 Four dimensions of trauma-informed asana yoga practice: intention, shape, tempo (pace), effort, keyed to the effect on the ANS.

to mitigate symptoms of distress, is the key to selecting the other elements.

2 The shape of the pose can influence the arousal of the ANS. Forward bending poses, in general, tend to raise PNS tone by releasing muscular tension, relaxing the spine, and promoting an inward focus (Coulter, 2012, p. 381). In the way I teach the full forward bend, for example, the practitioner releases muscles from the waist, and allows gravity to bring the torso closer to the legs, finally releasing head, neck, and shoulders. There is no emphasis on consciously shaping the pose. Backward bending poses usually have the opposite effect, stimulating the SNS by employing muscular energy, consciously holding the spine in a fixed position and, generally, maintaining a greater degree of outward focus than in the forward bends (Coulter, 2012, p. 324).

Prone or supine poses can release tension in the muscles by surrendering the body to gravity, and generally increase the PNS activation. Bilateral poses can raise SNS and PNS tone alternately, in the twist from left to right, fostering flow and bilateral balance. The twists also encourage a deeper exhalation, potentially increasing PNS tone. Side stretches can expand the space between the ribs, encouraging a deeper breath, which can increase SNS activation (Kaoverii, 2018). Standing poses can increase SNS activation. Research has also shown that postures utilizing a posterior pelvic tilt will increase PNS tone (Cottingham et al., 1988, as quoted in Sullivan, 2020).

In my experience, modifications of these poses will change the SNS/PNS balance, and each person's execution of it may have a different effect. For example, in standing poses, extending the arms overhead, versus keeping them at the sides, will generally further increase SNS activation. Consciously releasing weight into the floor may reduce it. In general, using a prop like a pillow in some poses can reduce the muscular effort, reducing SNS activation. The complexity of working with postures to regulate the ANS emphasizes the importance of choosing simple postures, and breaking down their execution into small segments of movement, inch by inch, with the client pausing to explore the experience, before moving on.

3 Pace, or tempo, refers to the speed at which the posture or sequence is taught. When a pose is performed slowly, PNS tone generally increases. The client can experience the movements, with their accompanying sensations, much more deeply. Those performed quickly usually increase SNS activation. As a baseline, it can be helpful for the client to demonstrate the movement speed at which they are most comfortable. The therapist can then instruct the client to gradually slow down or speed up the movement, depending upon the therapeutic goal.

4 Effort refers to how much force is applied to the movement, determined by variables such as the degree of tension in the muscles, the level of emotional arousal, the level of disturbance of the thoughts, and even the degree of concentration. The effort employed can change a movement from a PNS enhancer to an SNS activator. On a more subtle level, "asana is not merely a physical structure, but a condition of energy" (Frawley & Kozak, 2001, p. 33).

The effectiveness of these guidelines is dependent upon the client's experience, which varies from client to client. For example, while a forward bend generally raises PNS tone, if a client was abused in a forward bending position, the muscles which generally relax in that position could tighten, so the pose would become a stressor, and increase SNS tone. For this reason, a close observation of the client in a posture, and a continual commitment to checking in with the client, are essential ingredients of the therapist's art.

Maintaining ANS balance

Once ANS balance has been established, the following guidelines can help to maintain it:

1 Choose a variety of postures which energize the body, expand it, contract it, move it upward, or move it downward, to balance the five types of prana in the body (by permission, Dr. Marc Halpern, Ayurvedic Yoga Therapy Course, unpublished course manual). The NITYA chair yoga sequence offers these variations. For example, the cobra pose expands the chest. The forward bend is a contracting, downward movement. As the practitioner's torso folds close to the legs, it assumes a concave shape, and the shoulders and head release toward the floor. The performance of the whole sequence energizes the body (see below, Figures 3.4–3.7).

2 Include grounding warm-ups, such as noticing the points of contact between the back of the body and the chair; using the gaze to connect with the environment; feeling the soles of the feet in contact with the floor; and/or taking a few deep breaths while bringing the awareness to the parts of the body which move with the breath.

3 Introduce bilateral poses, such as half moon pose and the half spinal twist, which have the potential to upregulate the SNS when moving to the right, and the PNS when moving to the left, creating balance. Alternate forward bending (PNS enhancing) with backward bending ones (SNS enhancing).

4 Use invitational and interoceptive language. Invitational phrases such as "when you are," "if you like," "I invite you," and "would it be alright?" empower the individual to make their own choices. Interoceptive language, such as "how does it feel when," or "what is it like when you," encourage the individual to connect with the internal experience of each pose, which helps them to recognize and articulate their felt experience, on and off the yoga mat (Emerson et al., 2009).

From this grounded base, the client may be ready to experience a variety of hatha yoga chair poses, executed at a moderate, yet comfortable pace with a goal of connecting with sensations and regulating the ANS.

5 Practice eye movements. Eye movements are the first practice included in the Integral Yoga® Institute class. By moving the eyes, up, down, diagonally, and in a circular movement, the optic nerve is strengthened and the muscles attached to the eyes are exercised. My experience, both as a yoga practitioner and as an eye movement desensitization and reprocessing (EMDR) therapist and client,

suggests that they may also be related to our state of mind.

The work of bodyworker Stanley Rosenberg gives weight to this hunch by postulating a relationship between the movements and the individual's ANS state. He discovered that moving the eyes left or right, up or down, or diagonally changes the tension in the suboccipital muscles, located under the lower edge of the skull (Rosenberg, 2017, p. 193). These muscles influence the position of the upper cervical vertebrae, C1 and C2, which shift when our physiological state moves between social engagement, sympathetic activation, and dorsal shutdown. These changes of position influence the amount of blood flow to the cranial nerves, which affect the ability to socially engage (Rosenberg, 2017, p. 164).

Eye movements are also a key element in the efficacy of EMDR, a successful psychotherapeutic approach to healing PTSD, which reduces the traumatic effect of individual memories. Researchers have hypothesized various neural benefits of the eye movements used in EMDR, but have not yet identified the actual neural mechanisms (Calancie et al., 2018).

The wording of the eye movement exercises is included in the yoga posture script.

Using a top-down or bottom-up process

Another variable in choosing the most effective yogic intervention is a top-down versus bottom-up emphasis, as described in Chapter 1. In a top-down approach, the client would follow the teacher's instructions, in order to assume a pose. With an emphasis on a bottom-up process, poses can be expressions of the client's/student's inner state and energetic needs at the moment. For example, suggesting spontaneous movements may support the client in the release of muscle tension and increase blood flow to that area, which allows the client to be more present. The therapist can integrate both approaches, alternating periods of instruction with interludes encouraging the personal exploration of movement, with verbal cues such as, "what kind of movement does your body want to do right now?" Of course, some clients may not be ready for self-direction.

While a bottom-up process is less commonly supported in our societal institutions, including education and medicine, for example, both approaches meet real needs: the top-down approach for structure and direction, and the bottom-up for self-expression, enhanced interoception, nervous system regulation, and energetic healing. The guidelines at the end of the chapter provide additional perspectives on teaching a NITYA class which incorporates both polarities.

A sample posture and its benefits: the half-spinal twist

Instruction in the pose: For the half spinal twist, sitting with your spine straight, you are invited to raise the arms overhead and twist to the right, moving from the waist, up the torso, through the shoulders, neck, and head, ending by gazing over the right shoulder (Figure 3.2). With the left hand, feel free to grasp the outside of your right thigh. Place your right hand on the seat or arm of the chair in a comfortable, supportive position. You are invited to hold the pose and breathe, bringing your awareness to your entire spine. After the next exhalation, feel free to twist to the right just a little bit more, without straining. On the inhale, please release the pose, untwisting the torso, arms, and legs, and returning to center.

You can repeat the posture on the left side. To begin, please raise your arms overhead and twist to the left, from the waist, up through the torso, neck, and head. You can gaze over your left shoulder. Grasping the outside of the left thigh with the right hand, you can place your left hand on the seat or arm of the chair. You are welcome to hold the pose and breathe, focusing on your body

sensations. After the next exhalation, you can try twisting around a little farther to the left. Again, you can bring your awareness to the sensations in the spine. On the exhale, release the pose, untwist the torso, arms, and legs, and return to center. Take a moment to experience your body sensations and breath.

Benefits from the poses can vary from person to person. What is comforting to one person may be alarming to another, depending upon their personal history, current health condition, and the traumas the body is holding. Ideally, the execution of each pose will be a blending of top-down and bottom-up approaches, tailored for each client.

In the half-spinal twist, clients can experience many of the following:

- New body positions, which can encourage curiosity and exploration.

- The steady rhythm of the breath and heartbeat, which can be comforting.

- An intensification, and then release, of muscular tension, which can promote relaxation and reduce anxiety.

- A release to gravity, which can enhance the experience of feeling supported.

- A compression of the spine, which can result in an increase in energy flow, and improved circulation to that area.

- When done bilaterally, the twist may balance the tone of the SNS and PNS.

- The potential of an enhanced connection between practitioner and client.

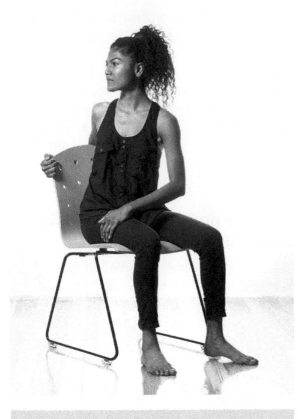

Figure 3.2 Half spinal twist, right.

The annotated chair yoga warm-up and postures script

The annotated version of the chair yoga script is included below (the non-annotated version is in Appendix 3). Written for the therapist, it includes the correct wording for teaching a pose, rationales for including particular warm-ups and poses in the script, and a description of additional benefits. The script can be particularly helpful for therapists who are not certified yoga instructors, as a starting point. It offers at least one pose from each of the "shape" categories which I have included: backward bending, forward bending, standing, lying (reinterpreted as resting for three breaths in the chair yoga script), and bilateral.

The poses included in it are a small sample of appropriate poses. As the therapist becomes more knowledgeable about yoga, and better able to teach it, they can offer the client a variety of poses to choose from which have a similar effect on the ANS. This approach is an alternative to relying on the same predetermined sequences for everyone. Here it is:

SCRIPT

The focus in chair yoga is to enhance your ability to feel your body sensations and to tune more fully into your breath. All instructions are only guidelines. You are welcome to participate in a way that works for you. Please discontinue the practice if you feel pain.

Please take a comfortable seated position with your feet touching the floor (*you can use a pillow or block under your feet if necessary*), your spine as straight as possible, and your hands resting on your knees or thighs. (*Posture, especially the straightness of the spine, will influence the flow of the prana.*) You are welcome to pause and take a breath. (*Even one breath can regulate the ANS.*) Notice the points of contact between the back of your body and the chair and the soles of your feet and the floor. (*Awareness of contact increases grounding, to counteract the tendency toward dissociation, and experience the body more deeply.*) You are invited to tune in to the natural flow of your breath, watching it as it flows in and out, and not trying to change it, for three breaths.

You are now welcome to do some arm breathing, raising your arms as you inhale and lowering them as you exhale. Please continue that for three breaths, on your own. (*This gives the client practice coordinating movement and breath and shows the therapist the rate of the client's breathing pattern.*) As you exhale, you may feel yourself sinking a little bit deeper into the chair.

Joint warm-up

(These are not yoga postures, but, rather, prepare the body for the postures.)

You are invited to rotate the major joints of the body, warming them up for the postures. You can start by rotating your fingers, then the wrists, in both directions. (Pause.) You can then move your awareness up the arm and slowly rotate the elbows, first in one direction and then the other, and then the shoulders. You can now let that movement go. How is your breathing? (Pause.) Making slow movements, as you inhale, you can raise the shoulders toward the ears. Then you can press them down toward the feet, exhaling. Pause for an inhale. On the next exhale, you can squeeze the shoulders together toward the center of the chest. When you are ready, on an inhale, arch the spine and bring the shoulders toward the center of the back. Then you can release the shoulders, bring your spine back to neutral, and pause to take a breath.

Now you are invited to move your awareness to the toes and feet. You may want to remove your shoes. You can stretch the toes, then rotate the ankles in both directions. Pause to take a breath. You can move your awareness up your legs to the knees. Inhale as you raise the right leg, and exhale as you lower it. Do the same thing with the left leg. Now, if you are able, on your next inhale, raise both legs at the same time, continuing to breathe. *(Holding with large muscles, like those of the anterior thigh, can intensify the experience of embodiment and strength.)* Hold them as long as you comfortably can (up to 10 seconds) and then release them. Pause to take three breaths.

You are now invited to explore the range of motion in the spine, first, on the inhale, arching it, bringing the shoulder blades closer together, toward the center of the back. Slowly continue this backward curving motion with the neck and head, raising them an inch or two. Then you are welcome to do the opposite, on the exhale, flexing the spine into a c-shape and curving the neck and head forward. Feel free to continue exploring these movements in coordination with the breath. (Pause.)

Now, bring your awareness to your waist. On your next inhale, begin rotating the torso, from the waist, in a clockwise direction, over the seated hips. What sensations do you notice? (Pause.) Now rotate the torso in the other direction. (Pause.) You can come back to center and take three breaths.

Moving your awareness up the body, you can focus on relaxing the neck. You are welcome to very slowly nod your head *yes,* only to the edge of your comfort zone. You can inhale as you raise

it, and exhale as you lower it. Then you can shake your head *no,* moving the head slowly from side to side, moving through center. Let your breath set the pace. (Pause.) Come back to stillness. Now, as you exhale, let your right ear tilt toward the right shoulder. Take three breaths in that position, if that is comfortable. Now straighten your head and let the left ear tilt toward the left shoulder. You can exhale as the head tilts and inhale as it straightens. You are welcome to repeat this movement a few times. (Pause.)

Feel free to make any other movements, to relax your body a little bit more. Notice any changes in your body sensations and breath as a result of the warm-up.

The eye movements

(This section of the script incorporates instructions from Rosenberg, 2017. With permission of North Atlantic Books.)

Lying on your back or sitting in a comfortable position (Figure 3.3), head facing straight ahead, weave your fingers together behind your head, supporting its weight. Begin the first round of the eye movements by inhaling. Keep your head still during this round. On the exhale, look to the far right corner of your vision. (Pause for three breaths.) Repeat this movement, bringing your gaze to the far left. (Again pause.) Now look upward. (Pause.) Next, look down toward your feet, and pause. Now bring your gaze back to center. You can rub your palms together briskly, building up heat, and gently cup your hands over your eyes, with your fingertips in your hairline, until the heat dissipates.

In the second round, take a breath, then again look to the far right corner of your vision. This time,

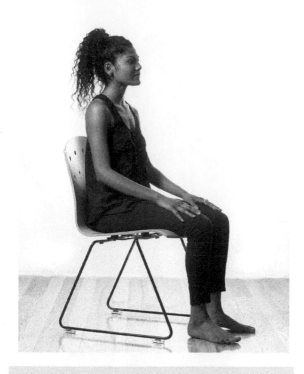

Figure 3.3 Simple seated pose.

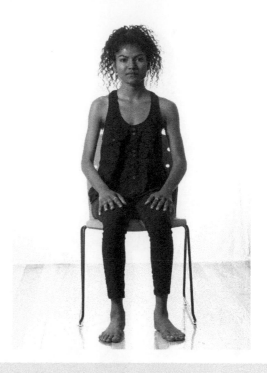

Figure 3.4 Seated cobra pose.

leaving your gaze there, turn your head to the left and hold that position for up to 30 seconds, or until you swallow, yawn, or sigh. Release the head and eyes, and repeat the exercise in the other direction, bringing your gaze to the far left, and turning your head to the right. Again, hold for up to 30 seconds, or until you swallow, yawn, or sigh. Release the head and eyes, notice the points of contact between the back of your body and the floor or chair, and the soles of your feet and the floor, and take a deep breath (Rosenberg, 2017, p. 164).

The chair poses

The first chair pose is a backward bending pose, the **cobra pose** (Figure 3.4). *(The backward bending poses increase SNS charge, because some muscular strength is required to assume and hold them.)*

With the hands on the top of the thighs, you are invited to begin to slowly arch the spine and neck, opening the chest and compressing the shoulder blades toward the center of the back, raising the head an inch or two and looking up. *(Opening the chest allows for a deeper breath and, possibly, more emotional openness, with greater exposure of the heart center.)* (Pause.) If you are comfortable in the pose, you can hold it, and take three breaths. (Pause.) If your mind is wandering, please bring your awareness to the point between your shoulder blades. You can do this any time the mind wanders. Notice the flow of the breath and your body sensations. (Pause.) You can come out of the pose by straightening the spine and bringing your head and neck back in alignment with it. After you have released the pose, you are invited to look around the room, letting your eyes go where they

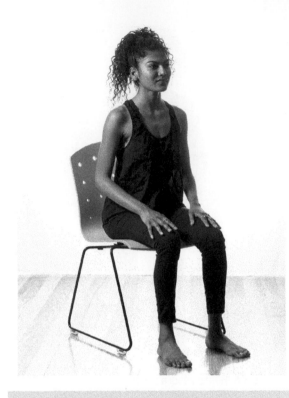

Figure 3.5 Forward bend, upright.

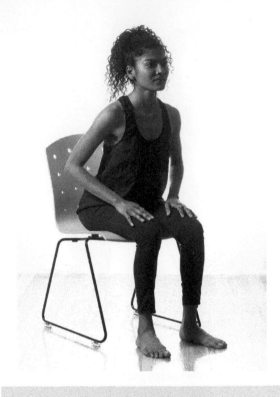

Figure 3.6 Forward bend, half-bent.

want to go. *(This exercise can increase ANS regulation by connecting the client more deeply with the external environment. It also disinhibits the eyes, potentially relaxing the eye muscles and downregulating the SNS.)* Bring the gaze back to center and watch the breath as it flows in and out.

The next pose is a forward bending pose, the **full forward bend** (Figure 3.5). *(Forward bending increases PNS tone because muscular effort is not required to hold the pose.)* Keeping the head as much in line with the spine as possible, with the hands on top the thighs, slowly bend forward from the waist, bringing the torso halfway down toward the legs (Figure 3.6). If you have a heart condition, uncontrolled high blood pressure or neck or head injuries, please hold the pose there.

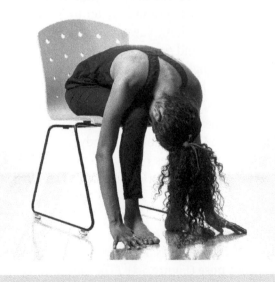

Figure 3.7 Forward bend, released.

If you don't have one of the aforementioned health conditions, you are invited to slowly lower your torso closer to your legs and, if you like, let your head hang (Figure 3.7). Or you can hold it in line with the spine. Hold the pose as long as it is comfortable, focusing on the natural flow of the breath. (Pause for 30 seconds or until everyone is sitting up.) Slowly bring the head and neck back in line with the spine and return to a seated position, with the hands on the top of the thighs. Please take three breaths.

We will now do the **seated half moon pose**. *(This pose balances the SNS and PNS, and opens space in the ribcage for a deeper breath.)* Sitting up straight, with the left hand on top of the left thigh, you are invited to slowly raise the right arm. With both buttocks on the chair, leading from the waist, lean the torso to the left (Figure 3.8). You can let the right arm arc over your head. Please hold the pose and take three breaths. (Pause.) If your mind wanders, you can focus on a point under the raised arm. After your third exhale, straighten the torso and lower the arm by your side. Repeat the same pose to the right by raising the left arm, bending the torso toward the right, and making an arc over head with the left arm, continuing to breathe (Figure 3.9). (Pause.) When you are ready, straighten the torso and lower the left arm. You are welcome to take three breaths

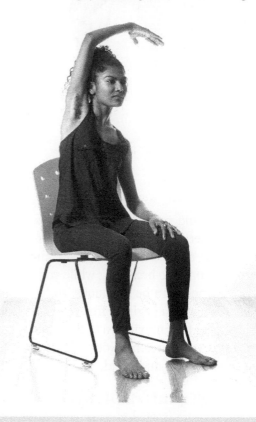

Figure 3.8 Half moon pose, right.

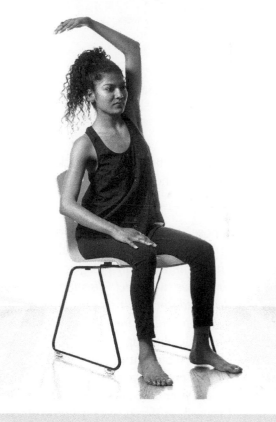

Figure 3.9 Half moon pose, left.

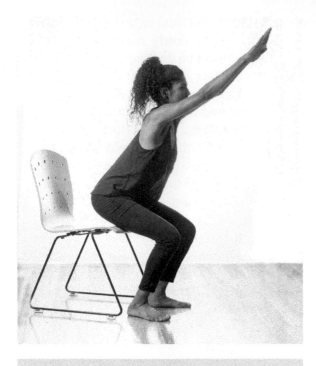

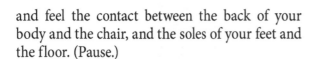
Figure 3.10 Chair pose, seated.

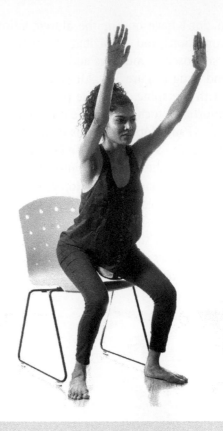

Figure 3.11 Chair pose, rising.

and feel the contact between the back of your body and the chair, and the soles of your feet and the floor. (Pause.)

The next pose is the **chair pose**, which can build strength in the legs and core abdominal muscles. *(This is an excellent pose for physically healthy individuals who feel disempowered in their lives, detached from their somatic experience, and/or want to upregulate their SNS.)* If you are dealing with a debilitating medical condition, or chronic SNS overactivation, you might want to opt out of this pose. If you are not, please put some weight on your feet and shift your center of gravity forward, as if you were going to stand (Figure 3.10). As you lift yourself a few inches off the chair, slowly raise the arms, so that the arms

are straight and parallel, and the palms are facing each other (Figure 3.11). Your head, neck, and back can be aligned at a 135-degree angle from the floor. Continue breathing while you hold the pose. This pose can be strenuous, so feel free to sit down when you begin to tire. (Have the client hold the pose for a maximum of 10 seconds.) Now sit and take three breaths. Notice the effect of this pose on your body and mind.

For the **half spinal twist**, sitting with your spine straight, you are invited to raise your arms overhead and twist to the right, starting at the waist and twisting the torso, shoulders, neck, and head

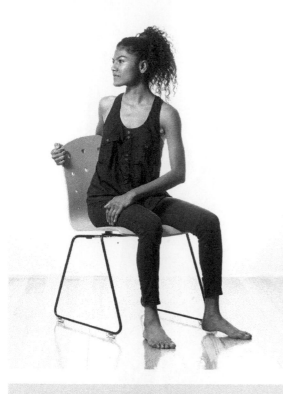

Figure 3.12 Half spinal twist, right.

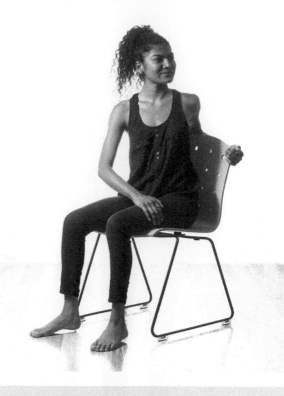

Figure 3.13 Half spinal twist, left.

(Figure 3.12). Gaze over the right shoulder. (Pause.) *(This bilateral pose also balances the ANS, bringing a fresh blood supply to the spine and supporting a deeper exhalation (Satchidananda, 1970, p. 64)).* With the left hand, grasp the outside of the right thigh. Place your right hand on the seat or arm of the chair. Hold the pose and take three breaths, bringing your awareness to your entire spine. (Pause.) At the bottom of the third exhalation, feel free to twist to the right just a little bit more. On the inhale, please release the pose, untwisting the torso, arms, and legs, and return to center.

You can repeat the posture on the left side. To begin, please raise the arms overhead and, starting at the waist, twist the torso to the left (Figure 3.13). Turning your head to the left, you

can gaze over the left shoulder. Grasp the outside of the left thigh with the right hand. Place your left hand on the seat or arm of the chair. You are welcome to hold the pose and take three breaths, focusing on your body sensations. (Pause.) At the bottom of the third exhalation, twist around a little farther to the left. On the next inhale, please release the pose, untwist the torso, arms, and legs, and return to center. Take a moment to experience your body sensations and breath. (Pause.)

The final posture is the **standing mountain pose**. *(This pose is sympathetically activating, due to the standing posture, as well as grounding.)* Please stand with your weight evenly distributed over both feet (Figure 3.14). Feel the entire sole of each foot in contact with the floor. As much

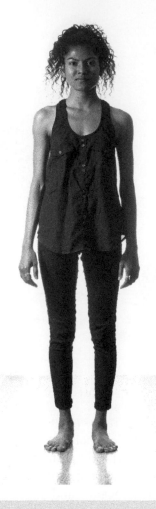

Figure 3.14 Mountain pose, standing.

as possible, align your hips and shoulders over the feet, and have the neck in a straight line with the spine. Now you are invited to bring your arms overhead and parallel, with the palms facing each other (Figure 3.15). *(Arms up is a more SNS activating pose.)* Take three breaths. (Pause.) Feel as if no one could ever move you from this spot unless you wanted to be moved. (This is an example of using a yoga posture to strengthen personal qualities.)

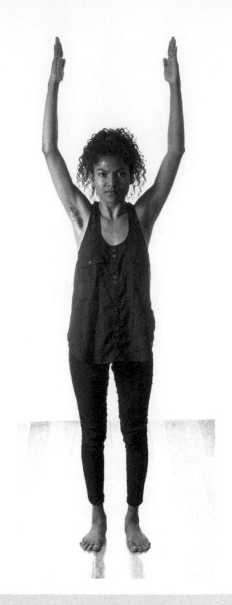

Figure 3.15 Mountain pose, arms raised.

After your next exhale, please release the arms, and take a comfortable seated position, with your feet touching the floor, your spine straight and your hands resting on your thighs (Figure 3.16). Feel the points of contact between the back of your body and the chair, and the soles of your

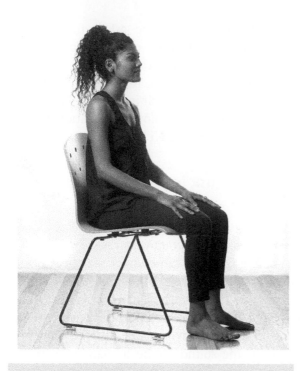

Figure 3.16 Simple seated pose.

feet and the floor. Watch your breath, for three breaths, and tune into your body sensations.

Notice if you feel different than you did before the practice. If so, note to yourself what the difference is. This is the end of our practice; thank you so much.

Thoughts about a mat-based NITYA class

There is a corresponding mat-based pose for each of the chair yoga postures included in this script, and their effect on the ANS would be similar. I haven't included photographs or a script for that class as the focus here is on including yoga in the

context of an individual or group psychotherapy session, for the purpose of using yoga to bring the ANS into the yoga zone. Using the factors of intention, shape, pace, and effort, plus the information on the functioning of the vagus nerve on the body, readers have enough information to evaluate each posture and sequence, to determine the probable effect on the ANS.

Applying NITYA hatha yoga to group classes

In a group class, a challenge for the instructor is to create a class which is therapeutic for people with different needs. In one example from early in my yoga therapy career, I was hired to teach a yoga mat-based class for an eating disorders day-treatment program. The class was evenly divided between what appeared to be very thin, hyperactive students and obese, lethargic ones. In a dilemma about what kind of class to teach, I chose a middle path, and taught a moderately active, SNS/PNS balancing class, which no one liked. The hyperactive patients thought it was too slow-paced, and the lethargic ones experienced it as too demanding. After a series of eight classes, the yoga class was discontinued.

If I was teaching this class now, I would meet individually with each student to evaluate their ANS needs, and teach a class with options which would work for them, based on the four factors described earlier in the chapter: intention, shape, pace, and effort. If there are a variety of nervous system needs, it may be necessary to teach two types of classes, individually or simultaneously. Each pose could be followed by a one-minute relaxation pose, savasana, where they are lying on their back, on their mat, with their arms at their sides and legs shoulder-width apart. This allows the ANS to re-establish balance. (To instruct chair relaxation, please suggest that the clients have their arms at their sides, their feet about shoulder-width apart, soles touching the floor. Suggest that they release their weight into the chair, and watch the breath, or focus on a place in the body, such as a point between the shoulder blades).

I would start with a posture sequence which could be done seated or standing, and which could accommodate different levels of physical comfort and flexibility. The same sequence could be rapidly paced to release muscular tension and pent-up energy in the sympathetically charged group. It could be taught slowly, and require less energy, for the depressed, dorsal vagus-dominant group. The eventual goal, arrived at slowly, would be to step up the pace for this group, while slowing the pace for the SNS overactivated group. A potential benefit for all students includes the experience of safety: of a predictable, quiet, peaceful, often beautiful environment where everyone is respectful, and has their own "safety zone" on their mat or chair. At the same time, they can experience being part of a group, and benefit from the ANS-balancing elements of some degree of social engagement.

Some participants may find it challenging to share the teacher's attention with the other classmates or distracting to have other students in the room. These situations can help give trauma survivors experience in being aware of their reactions. I recommend that participants have the opportunity to process their reactions in an individual therapy session.

In addition, you might try passing out squares of colored paper, with one color representing fear, one anger, and one or two more perhaps representing confusion or other common feelings.

The participants could be asked to put the appropriate color in front of their yoga mat or chair, if they start to have a strong feeling, or some other internal distraction, in order to maintain communication about their inner state. Please see the guidelines which follow for additional perspectives on teaching a NITYA class.

The use of music in a therapeutic group yoga class

I generally don't recommend the use of background music in a group yoga class, for two reasons. One is that it can distract the client from concentrating on their experience, which is the purpose of the practice. The other is that, due to the vagal nerve connection to the inner ear, some trauma survivors have difficulty distinguishing the sound of the human voice from other sounds. For those individuals, the addition of music could challenge their ability to hear the teacher.

Guidelines for using the NITYA posture sequence

The following guidelines are an original synthesis of nervous system-regulating hatha yoga practices, neuroscience research, and somatic psychology. While the level of distress and dissociation varies greatly from survivor to survivor, many of these guidelines are geared toward the trauma survivor who does not have good access to their body sensations. Depending on the presenting problem, NITYA might be the primary approach or else play an important role as an ancillary therapy in a mental health treatment plan. A keystone of this work is the quality of attention that the therapist may offer to foster the client's experience of safety.

1 Assess the state of the client's/student's ANS. After the assessment, a common strategy is to strengthen the functioning of the more dysregulated branch of the ANS, with the eventual goal of balancing both branches and re-establishing their natural oscillation.

2 Start where the client/student is. If they are curled up on the couch in a ball, that is their first posture. I recommend a gradual engagement with the body sensations, based on the client's capacity. Therapy could begin with as simple a movement as the bending and straightening of a finger. The client would then be asked to describe the sensations produced by that movement, guided by cues from the therapist, if necessary. The focus could progress to the instruction of a simple yoga posture, targeted to balance the ANS.

With an anxious student, it is often most effective to teach faster paced interventions, to meet the client's nervous system state, and to slowly moderate their system toward less agitation. The opposite may be true for depressed students. If a student is feeling lethargic, with low motivation, it can be most effective to begin with slow-paced movements and gradually increase the pace. This strategy will eventually upregulate the SNS, a precondition of ANS regulation. It is often helpful to have the student hold a pose long enough to experience its effects, but not so long that their attention drifts.

3 Demonstrate the pose, then do it along with the client. This approach may activate the client's mirror neurons, making it easier for them to practice it.

4 Emphasize that a healing effect of the practice comes from keeping one's attention on the movements. Moving with awareness trains the observer part of the mind to remain focused and gives a client/student more practice in identifying, experiencing and tolerating physical sensation. It also increases neuroplasticity.

5 Help the client/student to maintain a focus on the breath, in conjunction with movement. This can be a slow and difficult process for a trauma survivor, since it may involve experiencing uncomfortable feelings located in the abdomen. It can help to begin this practice by coordinating the breath with the movement of the arms, as in arm breathing, described in the annotated script.

6 Choose postures consciously, focusing on intention, shape, pace, and effort. Once your intention is established, offer the client postures from the appropriate category. If you are an experienced yogi, demonstrate several postures which have the desired effect on the ANS, and have the client choose their favorite! The more they enjoy doing a particular posture, the more likely they are to do it on their own, be relaxed in the posture, and experience a greater degree of regulation.

7 Suggest a point of somatic focus for each pose to concentrate prana and ground the restless mind. You can choose the point offering the most compression or the greatest sensation. An example would be to ask the client in a forward bend to focus their attention on a point between their shoulder blades.

8 When the client/student is ready, encourage him or her to work toward holding the

posture still for a period of time, in order to enhance the inner experience of the pose. Being able to do this is a sign of feeling safe, since it is difficult for a mammal to immobilize without fear (Porges & Dana, 2018, p. 63).

9 When teaching bilateral poses, instruct students to practice on the right side of the body and then the left, to activate and then calm the ANS and balance the prana. (There may be certain cases where it is preferable to calm and then activate, in which case, the practice would be to the left, then the right).

10 Unless the client is very lethargic, include a rest in the relaxation pose (also known as the corpse pose) for 1 minute or so between each dynamic pose. This practice is called "cyclic meditation" in the research literature (Telles et al., 2000). Resting in the relaxation pose between other, more dynamic poses, gives the body an opportunity to absorb the benefits of the pose, and to bring the SNS and PNS into balance. This practice has been the focus of research studies based on a statement in ancient yoga texts that suggests that a combination of both "calming" and "stimulating" measures may be especially helpful in reaching a state of mental equilibrium. Results show that the inclusion of both yoga postures and relaxation in a yoga sequence reduces SNS arousal more than relaxation alone (Telles et al., 2000). A similar study, "Oxygen consumption and respiration during and after two yoga relaxation techniques," was conducted by P. S. Sarang and S. Telles (2006) with similar results. This rest seems also analogous to the "settling" time built into the somatic approach to trauma healing.

11 At key moments in the session, particularly when the client seems particularly dysregulated, suggest that the client/student look around the room, letting their eyes go where they want to go. This shift allows the client to connect with the immediate environment, which can help to put them at ease when they find it to be safe; to relax the oculomotor nerve, cranial nerve #3, which is usually controlled, and therefore tense; and to foster a spontaneous experience of aliveness.

12 Use your voice and words consciously. The tone of the verbal interventions is an important variable in trauma-healing because a critical tone of voice could activate the ANS's defensive responses. Conversely, a nurturing tone can further engage the ventral vagus nerve. In my experience, the amount of verbal interaction while the client is in the pose is related to the client's safety needs. Some people feel safer when with a talkative instructor because the words give their mind something to focus on. Others may become distracted by the information, unable to focus on their body sensations and feel at peace.

References to the anatomical and physiological benefits of a pose help some individuals connect with their embodied experience, while they will confuse and distract others. For example, some students may enjoy the mention of the Latin name of the muscle which tightens in a certain pose and feel more connected to their physical experience with this reference. Others may prefer exploring the sensation without activating the conceptual part of their brain. The therapist and client can explore both styles and decide which one best serves them.

13 Use the same sequence of poses in each class or individual session, to increase the comfort level and familiarity with the poses. When the class routine is known, there is no anticipatory anxiety. This security can aid the anxious client in relaxing their muscles; experiencing their body sensations; developing a greater clarity of mind; and noticing the relaxation which follows. Once the client is familiar with a pose, they may be able to use it on their own as a resource.

14 Outside of the class or session, encourage students to make conscious lifestyle choices which will support their stability and growth.

Remember that while these guidelines are an excellent basis for interventions, they are only guidelines. Each moment with a student or a class is a unique event, and the response is most powerful when it is attuned to that moment.

Overview of yogic breathing practices, or "pranayama"

In the session, the client has been making progress in using calming chair yoga postures when she becomes triggered. But the therapist has noticed that the client's breathing is shallow, which could be preventing her from making progress in the regulation of her nervous system. Working with yogic breathing practices is the client's next challenge.

Breathing practices are the most powerful yogic interventions available to regulate the ANS. The yogic term for such practices is "pranayama," or "control of the life energy," the fourth limb on the Raja Yoga tree. This chapter describes prana on the gross and subtle levels; details specific yogic breathing practices that a therapist may use to help the client regulate the ANS; and offers NITYA guidelines for bringing breathing practices into a therapy session in a safe and effective way. (The terms "pranayama," "breathing exercises," and "breathing practices" are interchangeable.)

The overall value of yogic breathing practices for ANS regulation

Respiration is one of the few autonomic functions that can be either automatically regulated by the body or consciously controlled. The yoga tradition has made the most of this aspect of our physiology, offering diverse breathing practices to achieve specific effects.

While the biological processes of breathing are complex, the basics of this approach are straightforward: when we inhale, we upregulate the SNS, and the heartbeat subtly speeds up. When we exhale, the heartbeat slows and we increase PNS tone (Jerath et al., 2015). As mentioned in Chapter 1, this phenomenon is called heart rate variability (HRV). On the psychological level, HRV is a measure of resiliency and behavioral flexibility (Berntson et al., 2008; Beauchaine, 2001). The more variability there is, the wider the "yoga zone," and the greater the flexibility of the ANS response (McCraty & Shaffer, 2015; Tyagi & Cohen, 2016).

Breath awareness

If a client is able to sustain interoception, one way to introduce breathing practices into a mental health setting is through breath awareness exercises, where the client observes the natural flow of the breath without changing it. This practice can help the client to engage with their internal processes and sensations without having to perform, fostering an acceptance of what is happening in the moment.

This gentle intervention has additional benefits. According to Dan Siegel, a person with an unintegrated brain can access only a chaotic or a rigid response (Siegel, D.J. inspire to rewire, https://www.psychologytoday.com/intl/blog/inspire-rewire). Breath awareness can enhance the brain's ability to regulate and integrate its functions, potentially increasing its ability to focus awareness and control emotional reactions (Herrero et al., 2018). These enhanced skills can improve conflict and response monitoring (Pozuelos et al., 2019), and strengthen qualities such as insight, empathy, intuition, and moral judgment (Siegel, D.J. inspire to rewire, https://www.psychologytoday.com/intl/blog/inspire-rewire). This practice can also improve nervous system functioning by increasing the thickness of the myelin sheath, a brain structure which conducts electrical impulses through the nerve cells (Siegel, 2007).

I recommend several breath awareness exercises. In a seated position, the client can focus on the place in their body where they can hear their breath, and listen for three breaths. Next, they can follow the movement of the breath in their body, as they inhale and exhale three times. Another option is to put all of their awareness on their nostrils as the breath enters and leaves, for three breaths. If the practice is comfortable, the client may gradually increase the number of breaths.

As an alternative, in order to more fully experience the expansive quality of the breath, the client can lie on their back and breathe deeply. He or she can also lie in a prone position and feel the expansion of the abdomen as it presses against the surface beneath it. It is important to carefully observe the client's breathing pattern and degree of ease in the practice: some clients prefer to experience their breath lying down, while that position is retraumatizing for others. As the practices continue, the client may observe that the duration or depth of the breath changes on its own.

Another simple way to experience the breath is with somatic movement, through "arm breathing," where the client raises their arms when they inhale and lowers them on the exhale. This exercise grounds the client's awareness in the connection between body and breath. It also offers the therapist a visible record of a client's internal experience. Throughout the breath awareness practice, the therapist can monitor the state of the client's SNS/PNS balance by watching for the signs of arousal outlined in the first chapter.

NITYA breathing practices

In breathing exercises, in contrast to breath awareness, the breath is consciously manipulated. While the manipulations may be easy to describe, they can be physiologically challenging for the person who, for whatever reason, has lost some ability to move the diaphragm and breathe deeply. They may also be difficult for individuals with chronic physiological, cognitive, or emotional rigidity, because the practices can bring formerly inhibited emotional/energetic material into consciousness, and trigger ANS dysregulation. The upshot is that breathing exercises need to be introduced carefully and thoughtfully, based on the client's current capacity and state of ANS regulation. I recommend three practices – the yogic three-part deep breath, alternate nostril breathing, and brahmari, the bee breath – which are among the most simple to execute and are the most gentle catalyst for the ANS for most individuals. Annotated scripts used to teach these practices are included later in this chapter.

I have not included Kapalabhati, Bastrika, and Ujjayi breathing in my recommended breathing practices. Simply stated, Kapalabhati consists of a forceful expulsion of air through the nostrils, pushed out by the contraction of the diaphragm muscle, with a natural and spontaneous inhalation. Bastrika is similar, but the force is applied to the inhalation and the exhalation. I omitted them because of their potential to highly stimulate the SNS too quickly, without a moderating mechanism. Ujjayi breathing is a practice where the throat (specifically, the glottis) is consciously tightened, as a slow, deep breath passes through it. In my experience, it upregulates both the SNS and PNS, and therefore is balancing to the ANS. Sympathetic activity is upregulated by the effort expended in tightening the throat, as well as the strong mental focus on that area. The parasympathetic function increases because of the slow, deep nature of the breath, and the potential to stimulate the ventral vagus nerve, which passes through the throat. I see Ujjayi as an advanced breathing technique which should be taught by a certified yoga instructor.

Five dimensions of yogic breathing practices

I have identified five elements of pranayama practice to take into consideration when planning interventions to influence the ANS. They are intention, pace, depth, pattern, and nostril choice. I explore these interventions in Figure 4.1 and the text which follows it.

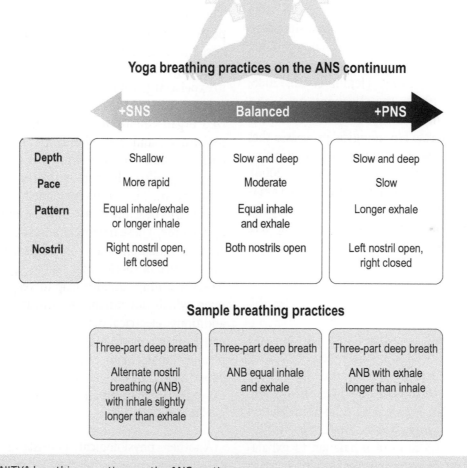

Yoga breathing practices on the ANS continuum

+SNS ← Balanced → +PNS

	+SNS	Balanced	+PNS
Depth	Shallow	Slow and deep	Slow and deep
Pace	More rapid	Moderate	Slow
Pattern	Equal inhale/exhale or longer inhale	Equal inhale and exhale	Longer exhale
Nostril	Right nostril open, left closed	Both nostrils open	Left nostril open, right closed

Sample breathing practices

Three-part deep breath

Alternate nostril breathing (ANB) with inhale slightly longer than exhale | Three-part deep breath

ANB equal inhale and exhale | Three-part deep breath

ANB with exhale longer than inhale |

Figure 4.1 NITYA breathing practices on the ANS continuum.

The elements:

Intention

As in the guidelines for choosing yoga postures, the therapist's intention is the key factor in choosing the best breathing practice to introduce. The Assessment Form, presented in Appendix 2, can help the therapist to formulate the intention.

Pace

Slow pranayama breathing techniques show great physiological benefit for individuals with ANS dysregulation. Research has shown that slow deep breathing upregulates the PNS, synchronizing neural functions in the heart, lungs, limbic system, and cerebral cortex (Jerath et al., 2006; Schäfer et al., 1998). Investigations have also demonstrated that slow pranayama breathing techniques moderate physiological processes that may be functioning abnormally fast or disturbing the homeostasis of the cells (Jerath et al., 2006). Another study concluded that the pranayamas which were most effective in lowering blood pressure, and therefore lowering SNS activation, were the ones which employed slower rhythms (Brandani et al., 2017).

Depth

Depth is related to pace, since deep breathing slows the pace of the breath. Because deep breathing compresses and activates the ventral vagus nerve on the exhale, a deep breath is a powerful downregulator for the SNS. While a 1:2 ratio of inhalation to exhalation is generally used, the most effective ratio may be a 1:3 ratio of inhalation to exhalation, a pattern which deepens the exhale as well as extending its duration (Bhavanani et al., 2016).

Pattern

As previously mentioned, as we inhale, we are upregulating the SNS, and when we exhale, we downregulate the SNS and upregulate the parasympathetic (PNS). We can use this aspect of our physiology to its greatest advantage in NITYA. The client can upregulate the PNS by making the exhale longer than the inhale, or intentionally increase sympathetic tone by making the inhale slightly longer than the exhale.

Nostril usage

The practice of pranayama highlights the therapeutic value of inhaling and exhaling through the nose rather than the mouth. The exception to this general guideline is in situations where one wants to expel a large volume of air in one exhale, which is easier through the mouth. The nose is a specialized organ containing structures to clean, heat, moisturize, and control the volume of air as it enters the body. To clean it, millions of hairs inside the nose, called cilia, remove unhealthy particles from the air. The "tunnels" made by the shape of the nostrils heat and moisturize the air as it travels up the nose. These narrow channels also allow the careful regulation of air volume, which facilitates the practice of subtle yogic breathing techniques. Nose-breathing can also help to keep the sinuses open, which can enhance health, as well as create additional electrical activity in the brain, which can improve emotional judgment and memory recall (Manalai et al., 2012; Zhou et al., 2017). An experiment, however, showed no effect on electrical activity when breathing through the mouth (Zelano et al., 2016).

Another physiological benefit of breathing through the nose is the increase in nitric oxide (NO) production, when compared to mouth breathing (Dillon et al., 1996). NO is an anti-inflammatory, hormonal, antiseptic repair agent for the body which can inhibit pathogen growth and stimulate the cleansing effect of the cilia, as well as a tissue dilator, which helps to keep the nostrils open (Lundberg, 2008).

Increased NO production has been linked to the practice of brahmari, a yogic pranayama done by making a humming sound while exhaling, which is discussed later in the chapter. This practice increases nasal NO production 1500% when compared to gentle nose breathing (Weitzberg & Lundberg, 2002).

Research supports the yogic understanding of the differing influence of the right and left nostrils on the ANS. Dr. Shirley Telles, research director of the Patanjali Research Foundation, developed her research on uni-nostril pranayama by reading a Vedic text, the Shiva Swarodaya, verse 105, describing qualities of the left nostril, and verse 123, which describes qualities of the right. Her studies show that breathing only through the right nostril increases SNS activity (Telles et al., 1994). In a review of pranayama studies, a number of other physiological and psychological effects of right nostril breathing were suggested, such as increased temperature and metabolic rate, both markers of increased SNS activity, and improved verbal performance (Shannahoff-Khalsa, 1991).

A review of major published studies concludes that breathing only through the left nostril will increase the PNS tone (Ramanathan & Bhavanani, 2017; Werntz et al., 1983). In a study mentioned above (in the section on pace), left nostril breathing, along with a slower pace, were the most effective variables in lowering blood pressure, and therefore lowering SNS activation (Brandani et al., 2017).

Recommended pranayama practices

In review, all of the following practices will increase PNS tone: a slow, deep breath with both nostrils open; an exhale which is longer than the inhale, ideally with a 1:3 ratio (depending upon the client's capacity); and a breath through the left nostril only. The opposite practices, including shallow, rapid breathing; an extended inhale; and/or right nostril breathing, will stimulate the SNS.

The center column of Figure 4.1 includes interventions which can be helpful to the client in maintaining regulation. Slow, deep breaths, done at a moderate pace, with an equal inhale and exhale, and both nostrils open, simultaneously or alternately, are recommended. Examples are the three-part deep breath, alternate nostril breathing, and brahmari.

The yogic three-part deep breath (deerga swasam)

The foundational yogic breathing practice is the three-part deep breath, done with both nostrils open, with an equal inhalation and exhalation. It is the practice upon which most of the other yogic breaths are built. In this practice, one breathes in the same pattern as does a baby: inhaling by expanding the abdomen, ribcage, and upper chest, and exhaling in the reverse order. "Coherent breathing" is a Western analog to the yogic deep breath, with a pace of 4–6 breaths per minute.

As previously mentioned, when an individual takes one deep breath, upon the exhalation he or she is compressing the vagus nerve in such a way that it sends a message of wellbeing to the brain, increasing PNS tone (Brown & Gerberg, 2012).

Additional research findings show that this practice improves psychological, neurological, and endocrine functioning, reduces perceived stress, and relieves negative psychological states (Pilkington et al., 2016, p. 98).

Dr. Stephen Porges noticed the benefits of deep breathing when playing the clarinet as a teenager (Dykema, 2006, pp. 30–35). He felt its soothing effect, which he later analyzed as the result of the slow, controlled deep breathing; the manipulation of the muscles around the mouth; and the mellow sounds; all promoting social engagement through their connections with the ventral vagus nerve. As I explained in Chapter 1, this nerve regulates the functioning of the facial muscles, lungs, and inner ear. Later, he recognized the relationship between pranayama and polyvagal theory. He says:

As a clarinetist, I was breathing. I was controlling the muscles of the face. I was literally doing pranayama yoga. I had no idea of that at the time, but I knew that as I practiced, it enabled me to think, enabled me to develop ideas and to control the state I was in.

(From an interview with Joseph Loizzo, https://nalandainstitute.org/2018/04/17/loves-brain-a-conversation-with-stephen-porges/)

Other possible effects of the three-part deep breath include:

1 Exercising the lungs, which brings oxygenized blood into the entire lung, promoting health and maintaining an optimal energy level.

2 Clearing the sinuses, which can help to stabilize mood (Manalai et al., 2012; Zhou et al., 2017).

3 Connecting with powerful emotions, which may be held in the diaphragm and stomach. (This effect should be carefully monitored for potential emotional flooding.)

Of course, some people may have difficulty breathing deeply because of medical conditions, a disordered breathing pattern, weak muscles, bad posture, or a disconnect from the emotions stored in their abdominal area. I would recommend requesting a medical evaluation for a client with a chronic, abnormal breathing pattern. Another potential difficulty is a feeling of light-headedness during the practice, because of a decrease of carbon dioxide (CO_2) in the bloodstream. This is because as the CO_2 level drops, the blood vessels in the brain contract, potentially reducing the flow of oxygen to that area (Yoon et al., 2012). At the first sign of this happening, the therapist should ask the client to stop the practice and reassure them that they are still safe. Ideally, the client will eventually be able to build the capacity to breathe deeply and enjoy the relaxing effect. All of these difficulties highlight the importance of using great care when introducing the three-part deep breath and modifying it according to the client's condition.

Alternate nostril breathing (nadi suddhi or nadi shodhana)

Alternate nostril breathing, also called nadi suddhi or nadi shodhana, is a variation of the three-part deep breath, done first through one nostril and then the other. In the practice of alternate nostril breathing, one blocks off one nostril, exhales and inhales slowly through the unblocked nostril, blocks the open nostril, and switches to the other one, repeating the procedure initially for three rounds. Once the client is comfortable with this practice, they can extend its duration with no harmful effects. This practice balances the activity of the SNS and PNS, targeting the ANS more directly than the three-part deep breath (Dhanvijay & Chandan, 2018). A study found that after alternate nostril breathing, activities that usually activate the SNS did not activate it (Telles et al., 2013). These findings suggest that alternate nostril breathing could be a natural remedy for anxiety and insomnia (Telles et al., 2013; Brandani et al., 2017). The caveat is that the degree of effort put into the breathing practice is a key factor which can affect the autonomic state (Pilkington et al., 2016). As in the three-part deep breath, I recommend that the client breathe slowly and deeply while keeping the effort low, if possible.

Interestingly, a research study confirmed that the effect of alternate nostril breathing on the ANS is determined by which nostril is used initially for the inhalation, not the one used for exhalation. A right nostril-initiated alternate nostril breathing technique produced sympathetic arousal, and a left nostril-initiated alternate nostril breathing technique induced the parasympathetic effects of relaxation and balance (Telles et al., 1994).

Brahmari (also spelled "bhramari")

One of the Sanskrit meanings of the word brahmari is "bee." To perform the brahmari breath, the practitioner inhales, then exhales slowly, with the mouth closed, while consciously making a buzzing sound in the throat, similar to the sound of a bee. A review of the research shows that the practice of brahmari can increase parasympathetic tone (Kuppusamy et al., 2017). It has also been shown to increase nasal NO production by 1500% when compared to gentle nose breathing (Lundberg, 2008). While one is practicing brahmari, discursive thoughts generally stop, making

it a possible intervention for obsessive compulsive disorder (Shannahoff-Khalsa & Beckett, 1996); Weintraub, 2014).

I would like to emphasize that, from a Raja Yoga perspective, no matter what the lungs and diaphragm are doing, unless one's mind is focused on the movement of the breath, one is not reaping the full benefits of pranayama. As in all of yoga practice, the deepest goal is to focus the mind, which calms and directs prana.

SCRIPT

Annotated pranayama script

Adapted from the Integral Yoga® Hatha Teacher Training Manual ©2017 Satchidananda Ashram-Yogaville Inc. Used with permission.

The yogic three-part deep breath

The yogic three-part deep breath is the basic breathing practice upon which the other breathing practices are built. It is composed of a slow, deep inhalation focusing on three segments of expansion: the stomach, ribcage and chest, and a spontaneous exhale. *(The inhalation increases SNS tone. The exhalation upregulates the PNS by stimulating the ventral vagus nerve. Together, the inhale and exhale regulate the ANS with every breath.)*

If you should feel uncomfortable in any way during this practice, such as experiencing lightheadedness or dizziness, please discontinue the practice, and let the breath assume its natural flow. These symptoms are not serious, and usually pass quickly. *(These symptoms are usually due to a drop in carbon dioxide in the blood, which is quickly increased when the breath returns to normal.)*

Take a moment to notice the natural flow of your breath. Watch the breath, accepting it exactly as it is, for three breaths. (Pause.) Now begin the practice with an exhale. At the bottom of the exhale, begin inhaling into the abdomen, feeling it expand like a balloon. (*This instruction provides a pleasant image through which to connect with a sensory experience.*) You can place your hands on the abdomen in order to feel the expansion (Figure 4.2). This is the first part of the three-part deep breath. The exhale should be done in the reverse order, exhaling from the chest, the ribcage, and then the abdomen. Practice on your own for three breaths. (Pause.)

On your next inhalation, breathe into the abdomen, and then into the ribcage, feeling the ribs expand out to the side (Figure 4.3). You can imagine that the balloon is filled with helium, and it is rising up to the ribcage. Again, you are welcome to place your hands on your ribs to feel the expansion, and exhale in the opposite order of the inhalation. This is the second part of the deep breath; practice on your own for three breaths. (Pause.)

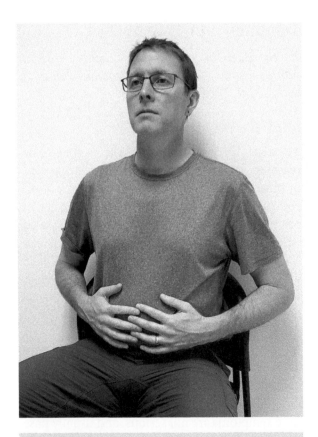

Figure 4.2 Three-part deep breath, hands on abdomen.

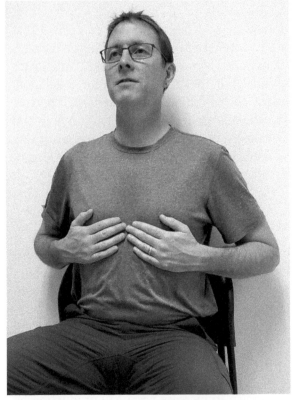

Figure 4.3 Three-part deep breath, hands on ribcage.

Now inhale into the abdomen and the ribcage, and bring the air into the chest, expanding the upper chest (Figure 4.4). Can you feel the collar bones rise slightly? Again, you can use the image of a helium balloon expanding to fill your chest. Place your hands on the upper chest to feel the movement. Exhale in the opposite order: chest, ribcage, then abdomen. This is the last part of the deep breath. Practice it for three breaths. (Pause.)

Finally, you can combine the three parts into one smooth breath. Practice that for three breaths. (Pause.) After the third exhale, allow the breath to

return to normal, and observe any changes which may have taken place in your body and/or mind.

Alternate nostril breathing

Alternate nostril breathing is the three-part deep breath done by inhaling and exhaling through one nostril at a time, then switching nostrils. To begin, please make a gentle fist with the right hand, then release the thumb and last two fingers. At the top of your next inhale, close off the right nostril with the thumb, and exhale slowly through the left. Breathe slowly and deeply, without strain. Inhale slowly through the left, close it off with the last two fingers, release the thumb, and exhale through the right (Figure 4.5). Inhale

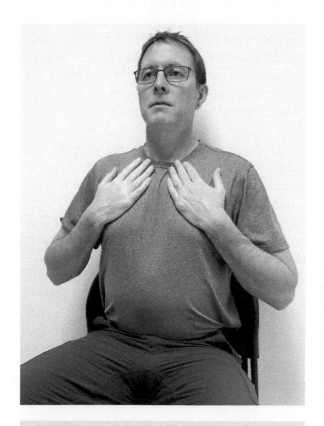

Figure 4.4 Three-part breath, hands on upper chest.

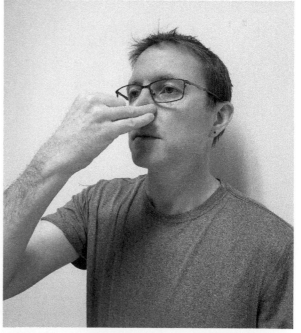

Figure 4.5 Alternate nostril breathing, left nostril closed.

through the right, close it off, and exhale through the left (Figure 4.6). Continue to breathe in this pattern, exhaling and inhaling through the same nostril, then switching. (Pause.)

After your next exhalation through the right nostril, discontinue the practice, bring your hand to your upper legs or knees, and let the breath return to normal.

Brahmari script

To begin the practice of brahmari, please inhale through both nostrils, filling the lungs completely. Then exhale while making a humming sound in the throat, with the lips shut and the tongue relaxed and in contact with the roof of the mouth. This practice

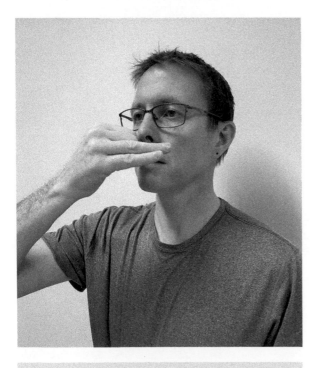

Figure 4.6 Alternate nostril breathing, right nostril closed.

vibrates in the head. Please note where you feel the most vibration (Satchidananda, 1970, p. 148.) You can also block your tragus with your index finger while exhaling to intensify the practice.

Pranayama on the subtle level

As mentioned in Chapter 2, yogic subtle physiology includes the nadis, the energy channels that interpenetrate the physical body and carry prana, life energy. Prana is inhaled with air, absorbed in the sinuses, and then goes directly to the brain through semipermeable membranes. It is also absorbed from the senses, the respiratory system and the digestive system. It then travels through the nerves of our physical body and the nadis of our subtle body, energizing them (Dr. Marc Halpern, unpublished course manual).

According to Ayurveda, the traditional Indian medical system, there are five subtle forms of prana, called vayus or "winds," which flow through the body (Frawley, 1997, pp. 314–315). They are prana, udana, samana, apana, and vyana, each of which describes a physical and subtle energetic process, and is focused on a different area of the body. Prana vayu is centered in the heart and brain. It moves inward and governs inhalation, the receipt of information, and one's mental state. Udana vayu corresponds with the throat and upper chest regions, and the functions of speech, which includes the ability to verbally express experiences and needs. It moves upward, cultivating enthusiasm and mental growth.

Samana vayu governs digestion, both physical and mental, and metabolism, and is located in the central region of the body. It relates to the pause between the inhale and exhale. Apana vayu, most present in the pelvis, moves downward and outward, and directs elimination, both physical and mental, including exhalation, menstruation, and all aspects of reproduction, and the ability to relax. Vyana vayu corresponds to the distribution systems in the body, including the circulation of blood and lymph and the fluids in the brain. It suggests a strengthening of one's ability to be flexible and open to change (Frawley, 1997; Sullivan, 2020, pp. 95–98, 171–172). In pranayama practice, the three-part deep breath fosters the balance of all of the vayus.

These energies work together. For example, on the mental level, prana allows impressions to enter consciousness. Samana prana assimilates them. Vyana prana disseminates the information. Apana prana disposes of the undigested waste, and udana prana fosters mental productivity (Frawley, 1997, p. 315). On a subtle level, one of the purposes of yoga practice, and particularly pranayama, is to balance all five pranas. Ultimately, trauma recovery and general mental health require the healthy functioning of these energies.

For serious spiritual aspirants, redirecting the flow of the vayus is the key to spiritual development. In advanced pranayama, practices are designed to cause prana vayu, which normally moves upward, to move downward, as well as causing apana vayu, which normally moves downward, to reverse its direction and move upward. These powerful currents of prana can then meet in the solar plexus area, and ascend the sushumna, the central nadi, to the brain, to fuel samadhi (Iyengar, 1978). Remember that samadhi is a state of pure awareness, branch eight on the Raja Yoga tree. (These specific practices are discussed later in the chapter.)

These are practices that go beyond physically-oriented therapeutic goals, and certainly beyond NITYA, into the spiritual realm. I mention this because I have seen advanced practices taught in beginner yoga classes, where the practitioners, and perhaps the teachers, are unaware of the vayus and how potentially dysregulating redirecting them can be.

What is Swara yoga?

Swara yoga is the study of the manipulation of the nostrils as a way to influence the ANS. One meaning of "swara" is the sound of the airflow through the nostrils (Bhavanani & Ramanathan, 2016). The interior structure of the nostrils contains a protrusion composed of erectile tissue called a concha (pl. conchae) (also termed a "turbinate") (Figure 4.7). In the healthy human, conchae engorge with blood, in a rhythmic pattern, in alternating nostrils. This nasal cycle, first identified in Western medicine in 1895, has a duration of between two and eight hours, depending on the individual (Keuning, 1968). The cycle is tied to the dominance of the SNS or the PNS. At any one time, the nostril which is not engorged is considered dominant, able to inhale and exhale more air volume than the one which is engorged.

In Chapter 2, we saw that the ida nadi ends at the left nostril and the pingala at the right. According to subtle yogic physiology, when the left nostril is dominant, expressing the qualities of the ida, the PNS, with its introspective, receptive energies, predominates. When the right nostril dominates, expressing the energies of the pingala, the SNS, with its externally oriented, assertive energies, is stronger. (It is possible to determine nasal dominance by placing a small mirror under the

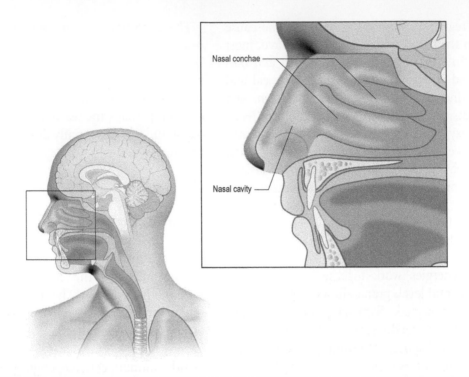

Figure 4.7 Interior of nostril.

nostrils and noticing the amount of condensation under each. The nostril with greater condensation is the dominant one (Raghuraj & Telles, 2008).)

There is scientific support for this assertion. In a review of pranayama studies, right nostril dominance was correlated with the activity phase of the basic rest–activity cycle, and with an increase in the sympathetic tone. The left nostril dominant stage was correlated with the resting phase, and with parasympathetic dominance (Shannahoff-Khalsa et al., 1991; Werntz et al., 1983). Swara yoga techniques allow the conscious manipulation of the nostrils, to activate the branch of the ANS which the practitioner chooses to be dominant.

There are several ways to switch dominance:

1 Breathing through only one nostril for a period of time, usually 10 minutes, will cause that nostril to become dominant.

2 Pressing under one's armpit, or squeezing a small pillow there, results in nostril dominance on the opposite side. This may be because pressure on the thoracic intercostal nerve, located between ribs number 5 and 6, adjacent to the armpits, can re-regulate the mucous membrane in the nostrils (https://www.yogajournal.com/yoga-101/deepak-chopra-7-spiritual-laws-yoga-challenge-day-1/). Alternatively, it may

be due to the effect of that pressure on the lymph system (Robin, 2009, p. 635–636).

3 Lying on one side of the body for 10 minutes opens the nostril on the other side (Davies & Eccles, 1985, as quoted in Robin, 2009, p. 634; Gottschal & Waal Malefijt, 2019).

4 Placing a piece of cotton in the dominant nostril for a few hours causes the opposite nostril to become dominant (Gottschal, & Waal Malefijt, 2019).

Balancing the nostrils

I mentioned earlier in the chapter that the three-part deep breath and alternate nostril breathing help to maintain a balanced ANS. Practicing the asana padadhirasana, the breath balancing pose, is another useful intervention in balancing the nostril flow, particularly when one or both nostrils are blocked (Figure 4.8). Here is the script for teaching that pose:

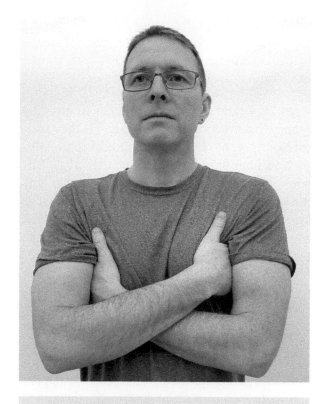

Figure 4.8 Padadhirasana.

SCRIPT

Padadhirasana script (breath balancing pose)

Please sit in a comfortable position.

Cross your arms in front of your chest, placing your hands under the opposite armpits, with the thumbs pointing upward.

The point between the thumb and first finger should be firmly pressed.

Become aware of your breath (pause); you are welcome to close your eyes if that feels right. For the next 5 to 10 minutes, take slow, deep, rhythmical breaths, until you sense that the flow of breath in both nostrils is equalized. Notice how that feels (https://www.yogajournal.com/yoga-101/deepak-chopra-7-spiritual-laws-yoga-challenge-day-1/).

Bringing pranayama into the session

The most important goal of the early stages of an embodied therapy is to increase the client's awareness of their body sensations. The therapist can begin by asking questions, such as, "How is your breathing right now? Is it fast or slow? Shallow or deep?" The therapist can also track the client's level of SNS and/or PNS arousal by looking at the physiological markers mentioned in Chapter 1. With that information, the therapist can choose the most regulating breathing practice.

An important element to consider in bringing pranayama practices into the session is the physical health of the client. Some medical conditions, such as high blood pressure, are exacerbated by stimulating practices. If the therapist has any doubts about the appropriate use of a particular breathing technique for a client, I suggest they consult with their client's medical professional, who can sign off on its use.

For readers who aren't certified yoga teachers, I recommend teaching only the three-part breath, alternate nostril breathing, and brahmari, with the prepared scripts (included in this chapter and in Appendix 4). Using the scripts included in this book as a guide, certified yoga teachers/therapists can write their own script. Eventually, clients will be able to take the breathing practice(s) learned in the session and use them on their own, whenever they recognize signs of ANS dysregulation.

Most importantly, the therapist/teacher can prepare to teach pranayama by doing the practices and maintaining excellent self-care, to have the maximum positive impact on the client.

Precautions when bringing yogic breathing practices into trauma work

I have included precautions concerning the use of potentially dysregulating practices, such as breath retention and bandhas, which are intended for spiritual development, as healing modalities, particularly with trauma survivors.

Breath retention

In my yoga training, breath retention was taught as an advanced technique, appropriate for spiritual development, but not for trauma healing. While it can calm a troubled mind, in my opinion, it was designed to still the movement of prana, concentrate this energy, and awaken the kundalini, rather than to meet therapeutic goals. This technique can have a destabilizing effect on the nervous system of someone who is not properly prepared to perform it.

Bandhas

"Bandha" is the Sanskrit word for "lock." Its purpose is to hold and accumulate prana at particular locations in the subtle body, in conjunction with breathing practices. The three major bandhas are jalandhara, the throat lock; mula, the anal lock; and uddiyana, the abdominal lift. These practices can be damaging for individuals recovering from psychological trauma, and I recommend that they not be practiced in the recovery process of this population.

Nervous system-informed, trauma-sensitive pranayama guidelines

The following summary of the NITYA recommendations can guide the therapist in using pranayama for nervous system dysregulation:

1 Choose a description of the practice that fits the client's world view.

For example, the therapist could describe the interventions as breathing practices, rather than calling them "yoga" or "pranayama" (Stableford & Mettger, 2007).

2 Obtain the client's permission to do breathing practices in a session.

3 Assess the state of the client's nervous system and the functionality of their breathing pattern. (An analysis of abnormal breathing patterns will require specialized training from a yoga therapy or respiratory therapy course.)

4 Practice pranayama and maintain optimal self-care.

5 Focus on helping the client become more aware of their moment-to-moment somatic experience, starting from their current level of awareness, and proceeding slowly.

6 Choose appropriate breathing exercises to bring the system into SNS/PNS balance, and proceed slowly. Altering a breathing pattern is a very delicate process for anyone, particularly for people with serious nervous system dysregulation.

7 Use breath awareness rather than breathing exercises with the reluctant or fearful client who has the interoceptive skill to observe their body sensations without becoming further dysregulated.

8 Suggest that the client inhale and exhale through the nose rather than the mouth, unless there is a reason to expel a large volume of air, in which case the mouth should be used.

9 Suggest that the client place as much awareness as possible on the flow of the breath. Arm breathing, described earlier in the chapter, could be helpful in developing this skill. If they have difficulty focusing on the breath, they can shift to the practice of the yoga poses, which usually have several points of focus, including the breath.

10 Do the breathing practices along with the client if you are able to simultaneously monitor their response.

11 Visually monitor the client's breathing pattern throughout the session.

12 Avoid any tone of voice or corrections which could activate the client's defensive responses.

13 Include psychoeducation about the effect of breathing techniques on the body's physical and energetic state.

Susan, a trauma survivor, is afraid of her rapidly shifting feeling states and feels hopeless about changing them. She is relieved when her new therapist explains why she is experiencing these shifts and that various yoga techniques can help her manage them. She emerges from that session feeling empowered, energetic, and motivated to begin this new chapter in her recovery.

The unknown is often frightening, particularly when it is happening inside one's own body. This chapter presents a map of the ANS's responses to threat, which has been termed the "defense cascade" (Kozlowska et al., 2015). This map explains some of the states the trauma survivor experiences, and serves as a template for NITYA-based treatment choices. We will also take a look at the related issues of dissociation, and the relationship between trauma and memory. This information provides a foundation for the use of specific NITYA interventions for different nervous system states (explored in more depth in Chapter 6).

Healthy autonomic reactions to threat

Life is most enjoyable when an individual feels safe and can function in a state of somatically-based non-defensiveness, the ventral vagal state (Porges, 2011; see description of this state in Chapter 1). In this state, the individual's responses are open and flexible, providing opportunities for physical engagement, emotional satisfaction, intellectual stimulation, and energetic balance.

However, all individuals are threatened by something from time to time. The vagus nerve continually assesses the environment for danger, using its faculty of neuroception, noticing signs such as others' tone of voice and facial cues. Normal physiological reactions to threat, often called "defensive responses" (or sometimes "self-protective responses" or "action patterns") are shared by all living organisms (Levine, 2015, p. 21). They include bracing, fighting, fleeing, and freezing, as well as several stages of deeper immobilization (Levine, 2015, p. 25).

In the aftermath of the threatening situation, the individual may also experience a variety of other symptoms, such as recurring memories of the incident, emotional numbing, and feelings of unreality. Within a short period of time, if the individual's nervous system is resilient, the ANS will re-regulate itself, and the symptoms will abate.

Some of the resources which promote resiliency include:

1 The inherently balancing effect of complementary processes in a healthy body, such as the naturally occurring alternation of sympathetic/parasympathetic activation, expressed in the inhalation/exhalation of the breath and the heartbeat.

2 The ongoing healing effect of interaction with other individuals who have regulated autonomic nervous systems.

3 The buoyant effect of positive experiences and memories.

If these resources are not available, their development can be an initial focus of therapy.

Chapter 5

The defense cascade model of the trauma cycle

The defense cascade model posits that when mammals, including humans, feel threatened, defensive responses unfold sequentially (Figure 5.1) (Kozlowska et al, 2015; Schauer & Elbert, 2010). When they are resolved, the resolution is also sequential, with the earlier stage surfacing when the previous one resolves. The defense cascade consists of:

1 Arousal. In this first, brief phase, the organism is alerted to possible danger, and observes the environment in a hypervigilant state. In this SNS-activated state, muscle tone increases (although there is little movement), as do heart and respiration rates. (In Schauer & Elbert's 2010 model, "arousal" is called "freeze.")

2 Fight or flight. If danger is present, the fight or flight response is activated. The individual mobilizes for action, exhibiting the signs of SNS physiological arousal described in Chapter 1.

3 Freeze. If the individual is not able to fight or flee, the ANS initiates the freeze response. In the freeze response, both the SNS and the PNS are aroused. The body mobilizes with tense muscles, caused by SNS arousal, accompanied by a sudden drop in heart rate and mobility, caused by PNS activation. This reaction is a momentary state, which either reverts back to fight and flight, or shifts to the next stage, tonic immobility, depending upon the degree of the threat. (In Schauer & Elbert's 2010 model, this response is called "fright.")

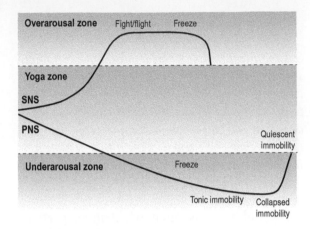

FIGURE 5.1 In this system, the first two stages are mobilization responses, initiated by the SNS. The third, the freeze stage, contains elements of both the SNS and PNS activation. Stages four through six are immobilization responses, the result of PNS-mediated dorsal vagal shutdown, which contain elements of dissociation.

4 Tonic immobility. Tonic immobility is the next step in the defense cascade, when fight, flight and freeze are insufficient protection from threat. In this state, the SNS shuts down, and the primitive, dorsal branch of the vagus nerve dominates the PNS. The individual may disconnect from sensory input from their internal and external environment and be unable to move or call for help. They may also experience coldness, numbness, reduced sensation of pain, uncontrollable shaking, the closing of the eyes, panic, derealization and depersonalization (Van Buren & Weierich, 2015). This dissociative response in mammals generally allows them to avoid notice and reduces energy consumption, instead storing it for a quick escape (Abrams et al., 2009). (This stage is called "flag" in Schauer & Elbert's model.)

5 Collapsed immobility. In the Kozlowska model, collapsed immobility is similar to tonic immobility, but the blood flow to the brain is further reduced, causing the flaccidity of the muscles and, potentially, the loss of consciousness through fainting. In that state, respiration and heartrate decrease, and movement ceases.

6 Quiescent immobility. In this stage, once the danger has passed, the individual is immobilized by a state of exhaustion.

NITYA offers interventions based on these stages of response, supported by a therapist who has gained the client's trust.

A closer look at dissociation

Dissociation is characterized by: (1) breaks in continuity in one's experience, along with unbidden intrusions of thoughts, perceptions and memories into one's awareness or actions; (2) the loss of the ability to access particular facts or control certain mental functions or (3) an experience of disconnectedness from one's self or from the environment, that may include distorted information about them (Cardeña & Carlson, 2011). These characteristics are a feature of tonic and collapsed immobility and, to a lesser degree, the quiescent healing period. It is woven into the fabric of overwhelming traumatic reactions, as well as being a separate category of disorders in the American Psychiatric Association's *Diagnostic and Statistical Manual of Mental Disorders*, Fifth Edition (DSM-5) (American Psychiatric Publishing, 2013). (The DSM defines "dissociative disorder," as "a disruption of and/or discontinuity in the normal integration of consciousness, memory, identity, emotions, perception, body representation, motor control, and behavior" (American Psychiatric Association, 2013, p. 291).)

Symptoms mentioned in the DSM include amnesia; flashbacks; numbing; depersonalization, which is defined as being detached from, or being an outside observer of, one's mental processes or somatic experience; and derealization, defined as persistent or recurring experiences of unreal surroundings (American Psychiatric Association, 2013, p. 272). Immobilization is often a replay of the original traumatic incident, where the victim was not able to physically move to protect themself (van der Kolk, 2014). It is interesting that various degrees of physical immobilization, a key feature of dissociation, are not specifically mentioned in the DSM-5.

From a physiological point of view, these symptoms can function as useful survival strategies which can help the organism to survive horrific experiences or great physical pain. If the dissociated state becomes chronic, however, debilitating psychological and physiological conditions may result over time, such as:

- Self-harm or mutilation

- Suicidal thoughts and behavior

- Sexual dysfunction

- Alcoholism and drug use disorders

- Depression and anxiety disorders

- Post-traumatic stress disorder

- Personality disorders

- Sleep disorders, including nightmares, insomnia, and sleepwalking

- Eating disorders

- Lightheadedness or non-epileptic seizures

- Major difficulties in personal relationships and at work (Mayo Clinic, 2017).

There is also a body of literature which looks at the transcendent aspects of dissociation, a controversial topic which is explored in more detail in Chapter 7 in relationship to yoga nidra.

Storing unprocessed traumatic memories

Neuroscience research reveals that our experiences are stored in neural networks in the brain. While most experiences are easily assimilated into the networks, the ones which are overwhelming are stored as fragments or traces, awaiting further processing (McFarlane et al., 2002; Bremner, 2006). Dr. Levine labels the memory fragments "implicit memories" (Levine, 2015, p. 21). (In contrast, explicit memories are composed of facts and events, which are available to our conscious mind.) This understanding of the way traumatic memories are stored clarifies the role of somatic sensations in healing. A traumatic incident may be forgotten, but its disorganized traces live on as implicit memories, stored in the body (Levine, 2015, p. 23). In somatic-based therapy, of which NITYA is a part, the client may have the opportunity to finish processing this implicit traumatic material as it is expressed through somatic symptoms and sensations (Khan, 2014).

Trauma-related diagnoses and their relationship to the ANS

Post-traumatic stress disorder (PTSD)

When the individual is confronted with a threatening experience, and their inner resources are insufficient to cope with the threat, the symptoms of the dysregulation caused by the experience can linger (McFarlane et al., 2002; Bremner, 2006; Sherin & Nemeroff, 2011; Flatten et al., 2004). In this case, the diagnosis of post-traumatic stress disorder (PTSD) (DSM-5, 309.81) may apply. Symptoms of PTSD are described in the DSM-5 as clustering around five themes:

1 Exposure to actual or threatened death, serious injury, or sexual violence.

2 The presence of one, or more, specific symptoms of intrusion associated with the traumatic event(s). Intrusion symptoms include flashbacks; a reliving of the trauma over and over, including physical symptoms like a racing heart or sweating palms; bad dreams; and frightening thoughts.

3 Persistent avoidance of stimuli associated with the traumatic event(s). These could include staying away from places, events, or objects that are reminders of the traumatic experience, and avoiding thoughts or feelings related to the traumatic event.

4 Negative changes in cognitions and mood associated with the traumatic events, beginning or worsening after the traumatic event occurred, as evidenced by two (or more) specific symptoms. These could include a persistent and distorted sense of blame of self or others; estrangement from others; a diminished interest in activities; persistent inability to experience positive emotions; or an inability to remember key aspects of the event.

5 Marked alterations in arousal or reactivity associated with the traumatic event(s), beginning or worsening after the traumatic event(s) occurred, as evidenced by two (or more) specific symptoms. These could be

irritable behavior and angry outbursts; reckless or self-destructive behavior; hypervigilance; exaggerated startle response; problems with concentration; and sleep disturbance. The duration of the disturbance, for criteria 2–5, is more than one month (American Psychiatric Association, 2013, pp. 271–278).

These psychological symptoms can be examined through the lens of the client's physiology. "Flashbacks," a symptom of intrusion (symptom 2), could be the re-experiencing of an implicit traumatic memory in the organism's spontaneous attempt to process and heal it. "Avoidance" (symptom 3) may be related to some degree of dorsal vagal shutdown, in order to avoid being further overwhelmed by the intensity of sensation and/or emotion. It may also be an unconscious strategy to avoid the SNS over-activation, which would result from re-exposure to the stimuli. The "negative alterations in cognitions and mood" (symptom 4) could be another reflection of dorsal vagal collapse, where the negativity is intensified by a low level of energy, motivation, and stimulating hormones. The symptoms of alterations in arousal and reactivity (symptom 5) all describe a dysregulated SNS response, characterized by the classic signs of SNS arousal. These correspondences give weight to the importance of regulating the autonomic nervous system as an initial focus in therapy.

Other stress disorders

Acute stress disorder

Acute stress disorder is a DSM-5 diagnosis (DSM-5, 308.3). The criteria and symptoms are similar to PTSD. The main difference is the duration. In this case, the symptoms typically begin immediately after the trauma, but persist for at least three days and up to a month.

The categories of symptoms include intrusion symptoms, negative mood, dissociative symptoms, avoidance symptoms, and arousal symptoms (Substance Abuse and Mental Health Services Administration, 2014).

Comorbid PTSD

In the case of comorbid PTSD, the PTSD is usually associated with at least one other major psychiatric disorder such as depression, alcohol or substance abuse, panic disorder, or other anxiety disorders.

Complex PTSD

Complex PTSD develops in some individuals who have been exposed to prolonged traumatic circumstances, especially during childhood. Complex PTSD, a diagnosis not yet recognized as such by the DSM-5, has been included in the World Health Organization's 11th edition of the International Classification of Disease (ICD). In the new diagnosis, 6B41, Complex Post-Traumatic Stress Disorder, diagnostic criteria includes:

(1) severe and pervasive problems in affect regulation; (2) persistent beliefs about oneself as diminished, defeated or worthless, accompanied by deep and pervasive feelings of shame, guilt or failure related to the traumatic event; and (3) persistent difficulties in sustaining relationships and in feeling close to others. The disturbance causes significant impairment in personal, family, social, educational, occupational or other important areas of functioning (World Heath Organization, 2018).

As adults, individuals with this diagnosis can exhibit behavioral difficulties such as impulsivity, aggression, sexual acting out, eating disorders, alcohol or drug abuse, and self-destructive actions; emotional difficulties such as intense rage, depression, or panic; and/or mental difficulties such as fragmented thoughts, dissociation, and amnesia (World Health Organization, 2018).

In this diagnosis, the symptoms are described in affective terms, rather than physiological ones. Yet the symptoms mentioned above seem to be classic indications of ANS dysregulation, and can be treated as such. Dr. Porges has noted that one's underlying autonomic state heavily influences one's responses to, and attitudes about, life events (Porges, 2009). Thinking along these lines, one can ask, what is the ANS dysregulation which accompanies the dysregulated affect? To what degree are the beliefs about self, and the ability to relate to others, a reflection of an underlying autonomic dysregulation?

A feature not yet written into the description of complex trauma is the potentially debilitating effect of microaggressions, which are, according to authority Derald Wing Sue, PhD, "the brief and commonplace daily verbal, behavioral, and environmental indignities, whether intentional or unintentional, that communicate hostile, derogatory, or negative racial, gender, sexual-orientation, and religious slights and insults to the target person or group" (Sue, 2010, p. 5, taken from Sue et al., 2007). Therapists can, and hopefully will, become aware of the effects of these subtle behaviors on their clients, and examine their own unconscious communication patterns and attitudes.

Yoga's greatest strengths in trauma treatment, with precautions

Strengths

As I have mentioned throughout the book, the practice of hatha yoga can help the individual gain a greater awareness of their body sensations,

which is the beginning of autonomic regulation. Repeated yoga practice can offer the client a lower level of ANS arousal during a challenge, easier maintenance of a positive frame of mind, a greater level of relaxation with less effort, and a faster recovery of dysregulated bodily systems (Gard et al., 2014). These features can give the client greater intimacy with their inner experience, and a powerful toolbox of regulating resources which they can use anytime, on their own, at no cost. As a bonus, yoga is normalizing and classes are found everywhere, as it is so popular in the culture (though trauma-sensitive yoga classes may be more difficult to find). Yoga classes and centers can also provide a social environment which offers an alternative to other, more sexually-oriented or substance-focused settings, which can be very supportive for individuals who are recovering from trauma.

Looking at yoga from a polyvagal perspective reveals that it contains many elements which foster social engagement, as well as supporting inner exploration, in solitude. If taught in a trauma-sensitive way, it provides an experience of safety. The student can experience a therapist or yoga teacher with a caring, sweetly modulated voice, and a kind face with relaxed facial muscles, radiating goodwill, as a resource. These features activate the PNS through the vagal response (Gard et al., 2014). If learning in a class, the traumatized individual becomes part of a group of peers with a similar, positive goal. If in a private session, they receive attention geared towards their needs. In both settings, they experience a quiet, comfortable, protected external environment.

These benefits are supported by a body of teachings that are based on centuries-old methods of self-realization, consistent with current findings in neuroscience. With this gestalt, the client has the opportunity to deeply internalize the experience of safety, which can slowly replace the history of distress with which many clients and students come into the practice.

Yoga philosophy teaches that, as their internal distress is resolved, a person can surrender into their true state of relaxation, peace, generosity, equanimity, and joy.

Precautions

While it can be a powerful healing experience, yoga postures have limitations and pitfalls for the traumatized person with nervous system dysregulation. At its worst, it can teach an individual with limited, rigid, patterned movements a different set of rigid movement patterns and practices, to which they can cling, blocking further embodied healing. For a traumatized person, this could be the outcome of a yoga teaching style which emphasizes external performance at the expense of an exploration of internal experience, or an adherence to a highly directive system with a sharply defined "right" and "wrong" way to practice.

Another danger is that yoga practices, particularly certain respiration and meditation techniques, will be misapplied, which can result in emotional flooding and retraumatization. Therefore, it is particularly important that the therapist be well-trained in a trauma-sensitive approach, such as the one I am presenting here.

Yogic philosophy can also be interpreted in a distorted way, supporting a judgmental, black-and-white view of the world (for example, "sexual activity is bad," or "extended fasting is necessary for spiritual growth"). I refer to this type of interpretation as "fundamentalist yoga." It encourages the creation of new polarities of good and bad, rather than helping to heal the polarities which are already present in the traumatized individual.

In addition, in my opinion, yoga lineages can misuse the concept of "ahamkara," the development of a separate consciousness in each individual. It is sometimes translated as the "ego," a selfish, limited part of the human personality, which holds onto negative patterns, such as selfishness, and lust, and must be destroyed. In my opinion, this view may be helpful to serious yogis, but it is psychologically shallow. I see it as a judgment on an individual's state of awareness which can misguide the individual toward self-hatred and/or self-righteousness. I prefer the more complex Western psychological models, such as Internal Family Systems, Ego Psychology, and Psychosynthesis, which work with "parts" (also called "ego states" or "subpersonalities"). Parts are unique sub-selves within each personality, with varying needs, beliefs, and behaviors. The Western models aim to identify, facilitate the acceptance of, and, eventually, integrate the parts, providing the opportunity for grounded, yet unlimited, personal growth. For me, the goal of that integration is an open-hearted, tolerant, peaceful way of being, which promotes a regulated ANS and can prepare an individual for the practice of the higher limbs of Raja Yoga.

In spite of these pitfalls, any yoga practice can eventually deepen an individual's somatic experience and increase self-awareness, especially if it is guided by competent psychotherapist or yoga therapist. When this deepened sense of self is experienced consistently, the yoga practitioner will have built an intimacy with themself that no one can take away.

The client, a beginning yoga practitioner, is looking forward to her first yoga-oriented therapy session. She has been frustrated by a cognitive focus in psychotherapy, which seemed to ignore the many messages she gets from her body. Enthusiastic about life in general, she is in therapy because she deals with anxiety and with an unusual amount of physical tension. This tension isn't relieved by exercise and hasn't been addressed by the professionals she has seen.

Applying the defense cascade model to NITYA therapy

One could look at the first four branches of Raja Yoga as having been developed in order to support the regulation of the ANS, rather than seeing regulation as a beneficial, but unintended, result. (I see the fifth branch, pratyahara, as a bridge between embodied practices and those which are primarily energetic and internal.) This chapter presents some NITYA interventions drawn from these branches, and tied to ANS states, which can support trauma healing. It can be helpful to apply knowledge of the defense cascade to the current state of the client's ANS, then choose the most effective interventions for that state, administered with skill and care. See the Treatment Planning Form (Appendix 1) and the Assessment Tool (Appendix 2), which can guide this process.

The NITYA approach to therapy

The application of NITYA to nervous system regulation in a therapy session is based on ways that yoga supports an embodied approach to trauma healing. This approach emphasizes the importance of the client's moment-to-moment somatic experience, which can provide a clear basis for choosing interventions.

This approach is most allied with a "functional/ developmental" style of body-centered therapy, which supports the client in discovering their somatic and behavioral patterns, observed in the present moment (Marlock et al., 2015).

Focusing on the content of the client's distress, and their personal and cultural context, are important also. Soliciting information on the client's life, including their personal history, current dilemmas, physiological state, and socioeconomic markers such as race, age, and marital status, can help the therapist understand the client's situation. This is particularly true since therapists are now recognizing that the experience of oppression, and the resulting trauma, are compounded by microaggressions inflicted on minority populations by anyone who has not examined their social conditioning (see section on microaggressions, Chapter 5).

At the same time, biographical narratives offer the therapist a story about the client which can be interpreted by the therapist's life experience and values, and can change with shifting diagnoses and cultural norms. There are many examples of these shifting norms, such as the removal from the DSM of the diagnosis of Hysteria in 1980, or the depathologizing of homosexuality in 1973. My hope is that working with a client's actual somatic experience is less likely to be influenced by the therapist's subjective stories and/or the profession's current hypotheses. (In writing this, I hear echoes of Freud's misinterpretation of his client Dora's symptoms as jealousy and repressed sexual desire, rather than the product of sexual abuse (Freud, 1905, in Gay, 1995).)

A different type of initial assessment would give the therapist a snapshot of the client's inner world, and an indication their capacity to be present. The therapist could ask open-ended questions, such as, "What is it like being here today? In this building? In this office? Is there anything in the office which draws your attention? If so, what is it? Do you feel physically safe right now? Emotionally safe? How does your body feel? What is the state of your mind right now?" If the the therapist listens carefully, and responds in an honest, empathic way, sometimes revealing how they feel, they can create a bond of trust. Of course, with some clients (and therapists), attachment wounds may get in the way of a bond forming, which is another important piece of information.

Out of respect for the state of the client's ANS, I maintain that it is important to gather biographical information at a pace which is comfortable for the client. This is particularly important at the beginning of therapy, when the intensity of being asked to relate their condensed personal history, in an unfamiliar environment, to someone whom they don't know, can be retraumatizing and dysregulating, and set a dissonant tone for the therapy which follows. I recommend, instead, inviting the client to speak about their life and current situation, while tracking the client's state of embodiment, as evidenced by the symptoms of dysregulation which I described in Chapter 1. The therapist can also assess the client's ability to orient, ground, maintain core support, and set boundaries. The demographic information and trauma history can emerge organically as the therapy proceeds.

Trauma-sensitive guidelines for working with a new client

1 Ask open-ended questions to gain a general awareness of the client's present moment experience.

2 Give empathic feedback in response to the client's experience. Notice how it is received.

3 Track the client's somatic experience.

4 As much as possible, foster an environment where the client's personal history can emerge organically.

The heart of the NITYA process

Signs of ANS dysregulation which emerge in a session can mobilize the therapist to gently interrupt the narrative, and ask the client what they are experiencing in their body. The answer can guide the therapist in their choice of a somatic intervention, which can refocus the client's attention on a present moment activity, such as taking a deep breath, doing a simple yoga pose, and/or orienting with the gaze. The therapist can also call upon the client's inner resources, such as moments of strength and/or experiences of safety, to contradict the distress. The point here is not to inhibit catharsis, but to teach the client to notice when their ANS arousal is extending outside of the "yoga zone," and to provide the tools to stay within that regulated zone.

These types of interventions begin to refocus the session from the content, which can be compelling but not productive, to the ongoing, primary work of ANS regulation. In this way, the therapist is focusing on the somatic experience of the client, which, though influenced by remnants of previous trauma, is alive in the moment, available to be changed, and usually a recurring pattern, underlying many stories.

Encouraging spontaneity

While individual needs differ, I also recommend that the therapist offer the client the opportunity to move spontaneously, in a bottom-up manner, to balance NITYA's many structured, top-down interventions. This will allow the client the opportunity to develop a stronger sense of autonomy and creativity. In support of this recommendation, Peter Levine says, "in order to recover … people need to feel free to explore and learn new ways to move … Only then can nervous systems reorganize themselves and new patterns be formed. This can only be done by investigating new ways of moving, breathing, and engaging, and cannot be accomplished by prescribing specific actions geared at 'fixing' " (Levine, 2015, pp. xv-xvi). In other words, nervous-system healing is an organic, involuntary experience.

Implementing NITYA in four phases

The implementation of NITYA therapy can be seen as a four-phase process for the therapist:

Phase One: Creating safety, which is described in its own section below.

Phase Two: Teaching somatic tracking. Once the client feels relatively safe, the NITYA therapist can use yogic interventions to slowly train the client to be aware of their moment-to-moment somatic experience, tracking it as it constantly changes. The yogic intervention can provide a container for the experience.

This is a major, ongoing undertaking for a trauma survivor (or anyone) who may have lost awareness of their body's messages, and does not know when they are tired, hungry, or tense. For example, a trauma survivor, John, was reluctant to engage in yoga postures, so the therapist asked him to walk around the room mindfully, and notice any tension in his body. After walking, he became aware of tension in his legs, of which he had formerly been unconscious. As he now consciously tensed and relaxed the leg muscles, he began to notice his shallow breathing pattern, which, with the therapist's guidance, began to deepen. When the breath deepened, he felt a surge of sadness, which he noticed and began speaking about.

Phase Three: Teaching NITYA skills. Once the client is aware of their somatic experience, they can be taught yoga-based skills and the appropriate use of each of them.

Phase Four: Taking the practices home. The therapist can support the client to use the practices on their own. Once the client is familiar with the signs of their ANS dysregulation and comfortable with NITYA skills, they will be able to use them on their own, at any time, to begin to reregulate their own ANS. This is the foundation for a comprehensive, empowering 24-hour-a-day recovery plan. With repeated, regulating interventions, the client may eventually train their ANS to move more quickly into the yoga zone.

Creating safety

"Safety" is commonly associated with an absence of danger on the physical level. An exploration of polyvagal theory can expand the definition to include social safety, emotional safety, and moral safety. Establishing social safety, which is related to physical safety, is an unconscious process using the faculty of neuroception to scan the environment to evaluate threat from people or situations. Emotional safety describes the degree to which a person can allow themself to be vulnerable and trusting. Moral safety comes from the confidence that there is a social consensus concerning right and wrong behavior (Bloom, 2013; Shea, n.d.).

This expanded understanding of safety can inform the delivery of therapy. The NITYA-trained therapist or yoga instructor can help to enhance the client's experience of safety through the use of basic interpersonal skills: a welcoming attitude; clear, respectful communication; attentiveness to the client's current state of body and mind; and, most importantly, a well-regulated ANS, the product of self-awareness and self-care. A well-regulated therapist is in a strong position to use the basic somatic techniques which are outlined below: resourcing, orienting, grounding, boundary-strengthening, and core support, and to offer co-regulation to the client, which is the regulating effect which one ANS can have on another. Many resources explore co-regulation in-depth, including books and posts by Beth Dennison, MFT (wecoregulate.com) and Arielle Schwartz, PhD (Schwartz, 2018).

Resourcing

Resourcing refers to the focus on any positive elements of one's experience: a positive relationship; a part of their body which is at ease; an inspiring dream, symbol, or myth; or, with some clients, on one's imagination, to fill in gaps where positive experiences are lacking. These inner resources can offer a buffer from the insecurity and emotional pain that often accompanies emotional trauma. Recalling even simple, positive experiences, like enjoying the flavor of a cup of tea, or

feeling it warm the throat as it descends, can help the client to overcome negativity bias, relax their muscles, mobilize ventral vagus engagement, and begin to break up limiting patterns.

Orienting

Orienting refers here to the ability to scan the environment through the senses (Levine, 2010; Hoskinson & Thunell, 2019). Orienting can be brought into the therapy session whenever the client's nervous system is triggered, to reestablish a feeling of connection with the environment. For example, the therapist can ask the client to visually scan the room for safety, connecting with objects, shapes and colors. If the client is open to non-traditional approaches, and it seems appropriate, the therapist can introduce pleasant fragrances, music, soft fabrics, and other stimuli to galvanize the senses. (Note: These interventions, which are soothing to most people, can be triggering to some. I recommend asking the client before introducing any sensory aids.)

Some traumatized individuals visually orient for danger, rather than safety, as a survival mechanism. If the client has this tendency, I recommend giving them time to do that, then asking if they found anything in the environment that makes them feel unsafe. If so, that is the material to initially explore. If not, the therapist can shift the client's attention to a neutral or positive focus.

Grounding

Grounding is defined here as the relationship a person has with gravity and weight as a stabilizing resource. To support the client's grounding, the therapist can encourage the client to assume a seated position and feel the points of connection between the back of the body and the chair, and the soles of the feet and the floor. They can then be directed to notice any changes to that connection as they exhale. Grounding can be further strengthened by having the client stand and feel the connection between the feet and legs and the ground. This can be experienced in the standing mountain pose (see Figure 3.15). Some clients may feel more grounded when they place their hands on their body in places that feel tense, numb, or unsupported.

Strengthening core support

Core support can be described as an embodied experience of strength and self-sufficiency. The therapist can begin this inquiry by asking the client to sense where their feelings of inner strength and power reside. This place is the source of their support. Once the place is identified, the therapist can work with the client to identify any yoga postures or generic movements which emanate from that place.

In the yoga tradition, personal power is generally located at the solar plexus. However, the location may vary from person to person.

Boundary strengthening

Many trauma survivors have "ruptured boundaries," created when their autonomy and personal space were disrespected. One way to deepen safety and empower the client is to explore the issues which arise in relationship to them. They can include the general level of privacy of the space; the placement of the therapist in the room vis-à-vis the client; the proximity of other students, if it is a class; the client's preference about engaging in direct eye contact, and any other factor which is important to the client (Emerson et al., 2011). Agreements can then be made which tailor the environment to the client's needs. The goal would be to create an environment where the client feels safe enough to engage, rather than be caught in fight/flight/freeze/immobility.

Using yogic interventions in conjunction with the defense cascade model

The "defense cascade," introduced in Chapter 4, describes the shifts in ANS functioning in response to an immediate traumatic situation. In the original trauma, these shifts maximized the organism's chances for survival. The cascade is reactivated when an individual is retraumatized, in the same order as in the original trauma. And as the individual heals, and the current state is resolved, the previous one in the cascade will reappear. For example, when the individual's autonomic system feels safe enough to come out of the freeze response, it will exhibit the symptoms of fight or flight. The eventual goal is to reverse the progression of the cascade until the ANS returns to a regulated state.

The following section describes the interventions and resources which are most appropriate for each stage of the cascade. The choice and order of the interventions in each situation can be based on a knowledge of the individual client's responses, as well as on these guidelines.

Guidelines for SNS downregulation through the defense cascade states

Arousal

GOAL: Assess threat.

Arousal is a brief SNS activating phase where the individual assesses the level of threat they feel. The therapist can help the client identify that phase and the sensations which accompany it. No other intervention is necessary.

Fight or flight

GOALS: Protect oneself until a feeling of safety emerges; discharge the residual ANS-generated energy.

Fight or flight responses are the result of SNS arousal in the face of a real or perceived threat. Below is a recap of the physiological changes which may result. In a situation where they are re-experiencing danger, the earlier the client (or therapist) can identify these changes, the more effective the discharge and recovery process will be.

- Sugar and fat enters the bloodstream, increasing available fuel.

- The respiration rate increases, raising the level of oxygen in the bloodstream.

- Heart rate and blood pressure increase, speeding the delivery of oxygen and fuel to the cells.

- Blood-clotting mechanisms activate, preventing excessive blood loss.

- Muscle tone increases, anticipating muscular effort.

- Sweating increases, regulating the body's temperature.

- The pituitary increases hormonal output to maximize focus.

- Digestive processes are put on hold, to divert energy to the extremities.

- The pupils of the eye dilate, offering the widest field of view.

- Short-term attention and alertness increase (Robin, 2009, p. 174).

- Blood is directed to the extremities, rather than to the organs and the brain, to allow for a fight or a flight.

The most effective yogic interventions for this stage are ones that will slowly increase feelings of safety, reduce SNS arousal, allow for discharge, and rebalance the SNS and PNS. They can include any of the following, depending upon the severity of the symptoms and the abilities and preferences of the client:

- Connecting with the environment through the gaze.

- Connecting with one's embodied power center.

- Performing a moderately-paced seated yogic warm-up, or any part of it, gradually slowing the pace as the client's SNS arousal lowers.

- Offering selected yoga poses that address the client's specific areas of tension and holding, emphasizing forward bending postures.

- Practicing the yogic three-part deep breath. Then, if that is comfortable, and the client is willing, adding more powerful interventions, including left nostril breathing, and/ or breathing with the exhale twice as long as the inhale.

- Exploring the practice of walking meditation (described in Chapter 8).

- Learning yoga sequences, to explore larger movements. If the client is sufficiently resourced, I recommend referring the client to a trauma-sensitive yoga class for an ongoing, more in-depth practice than can be offered in the context of a therapy session.

The fight response

The fight response is an expression of anger which redirects the blood supply to the arms and legs. (On a physiological level, anger is not a cover-up for hurt, as has been suggested to describe the emotional level, but a survival response, giving the individual the energy to take action for survival.) For example, in a session, a client noticed uncomfortable tension in her arms and chronically clenched fists, without an apparent cause. I suspected that she was experiencing a habitually inhibited fight response. To become more comfortable with the feelings in her arms, I suggested that she take any yoga posture that involved pushing something away. An example is a standing cobra pose, where the client leans into the wall and pushes against it until their arms begin to tire. By repeating the pushing each time that sensation is felt, the client can eventually become more comfortable with the sensation and begin playing with different degrees of pushing, perhaps experiencing emotional discharge.

Over time, with psychotherapeutic support, the client's ANS activation may decrease, and the activity may transform from a rigid, defensive somatic pattern to a more playful one. This approach works best when the client has the ability to keep their attention on the body sensations and emotions which are elicited moment by moment.

The flight response

The flight response, motivated by fear, also mobilizes the extremities. If a client becomes aware of the impulse to flee in the absence of any current threat, it can be beneficial for the client to work with the mindful movement of the legs in ways that will downregulate the SNS, in conjunction with psychotherapy. Individuals in a chair can press the legs and feet into the floor. The client can also practice walking meditation (Chapter 8), maintaining their own organic pace until it gradually slows, as the charge moderates. For those clients ready for a group class, there are a number of yoga sequences which involve movement, including the 12-part sun salutation, which will discharge tension from the legs.

The freeze response

GOAL: Enhance feelings of safety.

The freeze state involves a heightened activation of both the SNS and PNS. The immediate goal is to enhance the client's experience of safety, which will, hopefully, regulate and balance both branches simultaneously and allow the system to move back into fight/flight. To accomplish this, the therapist can foster the connection between the client and themselves, by establishing and upholding mutually agreed-upon interpersonal boundaries; using a welcoming and prosodic vocal tone, and, depending upon the client's tolerance for connection, breathing or making small movements together.

The therapist can:

1 Help the client strengthen their interoceptive skills, by encouraging them to connect with their body sensations, perhaps in a seated yoga pose, and by offering tracking support.

2 Suggest arm breathing, where the client moves their arms up on their inhale, and down on their exhale, for several breaths.

3 Focus on strengthening the connection between the client and their physical environment, by guiding a visual orientation exercise, and by encouraging the client to feel the points of connection between the back of the body and the chair, and the soles of the feet and the floor (Koslowska et al., 2015). The therapist can also help the client to foster the ability to make spontaneous movements, in order to release pent-up energy, and feel more empowered.

Tonic and collapsed immobility

GOAL: Upregulate the PNS and discharge the residual "fight and flight" energy.

The related states of tonic and collapsed immobility feature dorsal vagal shutdown, which slows or stops physiological functions below the diaphragm, such as digestion, and inhibits movement. Any effort to engage the client, and bring their awareness into the environment, can be productive. To work with this state, I generally suggest paying attention to any moment-to-moment, subtle changes in eye gaze, movement, facial expression, and/or breathing pattern. They present opportunities for inquiry. The therapist can begin introducing grounding exercises, such as feeling the contact between the back of the body and the chair or couch; slowly walking, noticing the connection with the soles of the feet and the floor or earth; slowly moving parts of the body, such as raising an arm; and, if the client becomes more regulated, performing more active yoga poses (Koslowska et al., 2015). Clients can then pause to notice if there is any change to their somatic experience, and/or their perceptions of the external environment, after each intervention.

Additional recommended activities for this stage include:

• Grounding and mild sensory stimulation, starting with feeling the points of contact between the back of the body and the chair, the soles of the feet and the floor (Schauer & Elbert, 2010).

• Exploring sense-oriented, SNS up-regulating activities such as to listening to music, smelling pleasant aromas, and touching soft textures.

• Performing simple motor activities, such as walking around the room (Schauer & Elbert, 2010).

• Exploring very small movements, such as bending and straightening a finger, which was also mentioned as an intervention for the freeze state, and verbally articulating the sensations experienced.

• Performing yoga postures at an organic pace, titrating the movement. This usually means slowing the postures down and experiencing every movement before going on to the next one. That could mean experiencing postural movement one inch at a time.

• Emphasizing backward bending poses.

• Performing the yogic three-part deep breath, either sitting or reclining, having the client place their hands on the part of the torso that is expanding.

• Experiencing the muscular contraction and release of a seated progressive deep relaxation.

Quiescent immobility

GOAL: Rest and rejuvenate.

The therapist can explain this stage to the client and give the client full permission to rest. No other intervention is necessary.

The progression of the stages of the defense cascade are mapped out in relationship to ANS arousal in Figure 5.1 in the previous chapter. Some techniques which I recommend for bringing the ANS into balance in each stage are displayed sequentially in Figure 6.1.

The sample interventions based on ANS arousal can gradually guide the client from the extremes of SNS and PNS dysregulation to the internal balance of the yoga zone. As you can see in Figure 6.1, the initial intervention in both polarities suggests beginning the treatment with an experience of safety and grounding, by connecting with the environment through the gaze. From that point on, the techniques gradually guide the client toward the yoga zone.

For the SNS overactivated person, initial interventions will be most successful if they match the client's energy level. To determine that level, the therapist can instruct the client to make spontaneous movements at their own pace. The therapist can then lead yoga-based warm-up exercises at the pace which the client has set, followed by a chair yoga sequence taught at a gradually more and more leisurely pace, with a focus on forward bending poses, designed to downregulate the SNS. This progression can end with the instruction of the three-part deep breath, with possible modifications: prolonging the exhale, and/or breathing through the left nostril only.

At the other end of the spectrum, the person with some degree of dorsal vagal shutdown needs to be met in a way that is comfortable for them. This process can begin with suggestions which don't involve much movement, for example, feeling the contact between the back of the body and the chair. Slowly, over time, the therapist can suggest larger and more fast-paced movements, adding the three-part deep breath and, possibly, a walking meditation.

Ultimately, the goal of this work is to maximize the client's experience of the regulation found in the yoga zone. The client healing from anxiety will know they have reached this yoga zone when they feel energized and alert, but not anxious. For the depressed client, reaching the yoga zone may feel like finding the extra inner push that is needed to get off the couch and start moving around. These interventions need to mobilize enough energy to slowly break through energetic holding patterns, and bring the ANS in for a smooth landing, into the overarousal zone, and then into a regulated nervous-system state, moment to moment.

Figure 6.1 shows the potential for yogic interventions to modulate over- and under-arousal, and bring ANS regulation toward the center, in the yoga zone. Interventions which can help to maintain that regulation include a variety of trauma-sensitive, moderately-paced postures; breathing techniques which balance both SNS the PNS; and, perhaps, a form of yoga nidra and/or embodied meditation which is comfortable for the client. Once the client learns these techniques and becomes aware of their nervous system state, they are capable of effective self-regulation.

Whatever stage of trauma healing the client is in, identifying the relationship between a body

Treatment goal	Technique

Goal
Increase PNS tone

Connect with the environment through the gaze.

Invite spontaneous movement at the client's own pace.

Lead moderately-paced yoga chair warm-up.

Lead a backward bending pose (e.g., cobra pose).

Ask client to focus on the natural flow of the breath.

Lead slow to medium-paced chair yoga poses, emphasizing forward bending poses.

Suggest, and lead, three-part deep breath, with modifications; longer exhale than inhale, or breathing through left nostril only.

Lead walking meditation.

Overarousal zone

Balanced SNS + PNS

Variety of moderately-paced yoga postures to promote balance and flexibility of ANS response.

Variety of breathing practices.

Trauma-sensitive yoga nidra and meditation.

Yoga zone

Goal
Increase SNS tone

Lead walking meditation.

Lead into moderately paced chair yoga sequence, emphasizing backward bending.

Lead moderately paced yoga warm-up.

Instruct three-part deep breath. Add chair cobra pose while performing breath.

Lead slow, small movements, like raising and lowering of arms in rhythm with the natural breath.

Lead grounding through feeling the contact between the back of the body and the chair, bottom of the feet and the floor.

Suggest connecting with the environment through the gaze.

Underarousal zone

Figure 6.1 Sample interventions based on ANS arousal.

sensation, an accompanying emotion, and a spontaneous thought or image can give meaning to the sensation. It can also provide material for the client to work with. For example, a therapy client, Bill, may begin to feel tightness in his throat (sensation), but not know why. He can then be encouraged by the therapist to practice a yoga technique, such as brahmari, which works to release throat tension by making vocalizations. Bill is surprised when he makes this sound, and is then overwhelmed by a feeling of helplessness, and starts to cry. Bill then remembers his father's mocking smile when, as a child, he tried to sing. This memory opens up a new avenue for him, that of healing his relationship with his father (meaning).

The value of slowing down the process

As mentioned in Chapter 1, the intensity of a traumatic experience can overpower the individual's ability to process it in the neo-cortex (Levine, 2015, p. 55). It can be stored instead as memory fragments and body tensions, awaiting complete processing. The unfiltered experience of these fragments could open a torrent of sensations, memories, and emotions which send the client into the overarousal or immobilization zones of the NITYA Healing Chart. In order to be regulating, these experiences need to be slowed down and experienced in small segments, or "titrated," with sufficient safety in place, in order to avoid retraumatization (Levine, 2010). Eventually, this experience of titration can train the traumatized individual to self-titrate when they are overwhelmed.

For example, if a client, Sam, is telling the story of having been the victim of an assault, and begins to re-experience the fear generated by the original incident, the retelling may overwhelm him, leaving him shaken and exhausted. If the therapist stops the narrative and redirects the client's attention to a resource each time the story begins to send his ANS outside of the window of tolerance (WOT), Sam may eventually notice the early warning signs of retraumatization. He can then slow down the retelling of the story, drawing on resources such as looking at a friendly face, or taking a deep breath, to restore a feeling of safety. He may then feel safe enough to experience a physical or emotional discharge of that bit of the trauma, which is the next step forward in healing. This process can help to re-program the ANS onto a more consistently regulated track.

Examples of physical discharge are trembling or vibration; as gentle fasciculations (muscle twitches) and/or changes in skin temperature; and as "micro-movements" (Levine, 2010, p. 93). Other physiological reactions include tingling, warmth, vibrations or trembling, expanded breathing, coughing/throat clearing, release of phlegm, crying, laughing, burping/stomach gurgling, itching, yawning, cooling, and clearing of sinuses. These releases can be observed in a body-oriented psychotherapy session; they also happen in yoga practice. Other examples of emotional discharge are sobbing, crying, yelling, and moaning (Miller-Karas, 2015).

When the client is regulated enough to tolerate some distress, as previously mentioned, the therapist can titrate yoga postures by suggesting that they be performed an inch at a time, slowing them down, and giving the client time to notice the body sensations and/or breathing patterns which are present, as well as any other information which may reveal itself. Practicing this way allows every nuanced sensation to be felt, whether it is pleasant or uncomfortable, further yoking the client's awareness of body sensations, thoughts, images, memories, and emotions. As Peter Levine says, "In order to unravel this tangle of fear and paralysis, we must be able to voluntarily contact and experience those frightening physical sensations; we must be able to confront them long enough for them to shift and change" (Levine, 2010, p. 74).

If the client is immobilized, in some degree of dorsal vagus shutdown, a different strategy is necessary. Over time, after experiencing slower-paced interventions and building resources over many sessions, the client can be encouraged to move more rapidly and/or breathe more deeply, until the ANS charge builds enough for them to experience their sensations, emotions, and/or memories more fully, while remaining comfortable in their body and in the safety of the yoga zone. Ideally, they may feel body sensations such as increasing strength in the upper body, a surge of energy in the arms, and a deeper grounding of the back of the body into the chair, signs that the client's full range of responses is being reclaimed.

Putting various trauma-sensitive interventions together

The following example uses chair yoga postures, three-part deep breathing, grounding, and boundary strengthening for the individual. (This is a very condensed account of the progress of therapy.)

A female client, Betty, comes into an initial session with a psychotherapist, T., to deal with chronic insomnia and anxiety, symptoms of past trauma. She walks in tentatively, displaying tense musculature and small, furtive movements, surveying the room with her gaze. T. notes that the client is most likely in the initial arousal phase of the defense cascade. T. then encourages Betty's self-empowerment by asking her if she is comfortable with the distance between herself and T., and the angle at which they sit. Betty cautiously asks T. to move back a bit and angle her chair, so that they are not facing each other directly.

T. then invites Betty to look around the room and more slowly connect visually with the objects which draw her attention. After doing that without experiencing additional arousal, T. suggests that she notice the natural flow of her breath. She does that, and seems to become more tense. She then begins talking about why she is there. T. pays attention to the body sensations which arise as she speaks. As Betty speaks, her SNS arousal increases, and she has difficulty sitting still. (Client is likely experiencing a fight/flight response.) At this point, T. asks her to feel the contact between the back of her body and the chair, and the soles of her feet and the floor, and then take a breath. As Betty begins to release to gravity, her muscles relax. They repeat this scenario several times during the session, with Betty speaking and T. instructing her to feel the contact and breathe. As the session ends, Betty seems to be in a mild state of fight/flight. At that point, T. suggests that she look around the room at objects that she likes. Betty does that, and seems to relax.

In the following session, Betty seems more sure of herself as she walks into the room, with more flowing movements. She tells T. that she is starting to feel comfortable being with him. Hearing this, T. is encouraged that Betty is ready for another intervention. After talking for a few minutes, T. asks her to stand up and assume the standing mountain pose, feeling the contact between the soles of her feet on the floor, and the support of her legs. When Betty does this, she notices increased muscular tension in her legs, a sign of a mild flight response. As this process continues, she experiences some trembling in the legs, which is a sign of the release of an old pattern of trauma held in the body.

To heighten a full-body experience, the therapist can encourage Betty to consciously tense and release the large muscles of the thighs, then notice any response. Betty can easily tense them but has some difficulty with release. After taking some time for Betty to notice her body sensations, T. asks her to assume a yoga posture which requires muscular strength in the legs, such as the chair pose. Again, she feels trembling, a sign of more release. As the sessions continue, Betty becomes more able to report on her body sensations and to focus on the flow of her breath, without leaving the yoga zone. She reports that the frequency of her insomnia also decreases. She is slowly moving out of fight or flight, and into nervous system regulation.

The therapeutic path is less clear for the individual who regularly shifts back and forth from state to state in the cascade, or experiences two states at once. In cases like this, it is particularly important to carefully observe the client's somatic state, and ask questions to ascertain what is happening in the moment. For example, if the therapist observes the client taking a spontaneous deep breath, and exhaling with a sigh, he or she could bring the client's attention to that exhale and sensitively ask whether they were aware of it. If so, the therapist could ask questions like, "what did it feel like to breathe deeply, and then sigh? What were you thinking at the time? Feeling? Did you feel differently afterwards?" The intention in asking is to help the client develop interoception, and to help the therapist choose the most effective intervention. The NITYA approach can be used

in couple's therapy, also. In that mode, I would take a step back from intensely tracking each client's nervous system state, to first offer them psychoeducation, in cluding a basic description of the ANS and polyvagal theory.

The goals would be to help couples to:

1 Understand what is happening in their own nervous system when they feel threatened.

2 Understand how they can help each other through the power of social engagement.

3 Learn simple yogic interventions which they can use individually, and together, to re-regulate themselves.

This physiological approach could become a different lens through which to understand what is happening in the relationship, which could result in more mutual empathy. It could reduce blame, and minimize guilt. The therapist can help the individuals identify their state in the session, moment to moment, which is the best teaching tool.

Taking the techniques home

As I have mentioned, the eventual goal of the NITYA interventions is for the client to recognize when their ANS is becoming unbalanced, and to use them on their own, outside of the therapy session. There are a number of ways the therapist can support the client in doing this, and a number of actions the client can take, to make that goal easier to accomplish:

• The client can keep a journal of their experience of when their ANS is dysregulated and what action they took. The therapist and client can review it together and appreciate the client's activity while possibly brainstorming additional options.

- The therapist and client can create, and practice, a protocol of NITYA interventions and of resources to use in specific dysregulated situations.

- Either the client or the therapist can make an audio recording of the interventions, and the client can play it when they need to address their dysregulation.

- The client can create and practice a routine of yoga and/or movement activities on their own to help them to maintain ANS regulation and body awareness.

- The client can participate regularly in a trauma-sensitive yoga class, and share their experience with the therapist, including moments of joy and of discomfort.

- The client can make a commitment to a lifestyle which fosters ANS balance.

Assessment tool and treatment plan for bringing NITYA into mental health care

Below are some key assessment questions which will help in treatment planning (also see the blank treatment planning form in Appendix 1 and the assessment form in Appendix 2):

1 Is the client open to a somatic intervention?

   Make sure that the client is open to a somatic intervention before introducing one. It is important that the client be on board with the intervention and invested in its success.

2 What is your rationale for bringing NITYA interventions into the session?

   A planful approach usually brings the best results. While research supports the use of yoga for emotional trauma, anxiety, depression, and other conditions, a somatic intervention may not be the best choice for every issue a client presents. It is useful to determine your particular goals for using this type of intervention with each case.

3 Does the client have any medical condition, or is he or she taking any medication, which should be taken into consideration when creating a NITYA-influenced plan?

   Since certain yogic interventions are contraindicated for some medical conditions, while others are recommended, it is beneficial to have current information on the state of the client's health. I recommend requiring a recent medical report (not more than six months old) before initiating a NITYA-informed treatment plan. You may also want to seek the doctor's approval for specific yogic interventions.

4 Of the four dimensions of heath (physical, mental, emotional, and energetic/spiritual), which are strong? Which are underdeveloped?

   After establishing the client's trust, it could be helpful to gradually shift the focus from the areas which are already strong to those which are underdeveloped.

5 What is your analysis of the ANS balance in the client (SNS/PNS overactivation; underactivation; both; no imbalance)?

6 What is the pattern of that client's defense cascade? Do they move through several stages when narrating a difficult experience, or do they remain in one of the stages?

As part of your assessment, you can use your observation skills as well as the client's information about the symptoms.

7 Can you address symptoms with specific interventions?

A solid treatment plan can be built by matching interventions with specific symptoms. Make a list of the symptoms which you would like to address, and NITYA-based interventions to use with each. You may use these as guidelines but be open to new options.

The branches of Raja Yoga, presented in Chapter 1, form a solid structure for choosing interventions to meet treatment plan goals. After assessing any health-related restrictions on the client's practice, filling in the optimal interventions in the blanks will form a basis for a Raja Yoga-based treatment plan:

1 Moral/ethical practices. (Is the client acting in ways that will hurt themself or others?)_____

2 Physical interventions. (How aware is the client of their body sensations? If they don't have this awareness, I recommend focusing on slow, small body movements, like bending a finger, before introducing postures. Is the client ready to track their somatic experience through time? If so, which postures does the therapist recommend for that client, based on the state of the client's defense cascade?)

_____

3 Breathing practices. (Is the client able to track the movement of the breath? If not, I would recommend exploring breath awareness before teaching any breathing practices. Is the client grounded enough to engage in yogic breathing practices? If so, which practices would you recommend?)

_____

4 Deep relaxation/yoga nidra. (For the progressive deep relaxation: Does the client experience significant muscle tension? For the practices which follow: Does the client feel safe and resourced enough to surrender to their inner experience? If they feel uncomfortable, at which stage of the practice does that begin? How do they feel after the practice?)

_____

5 Concentration and meditation. (Is the client interested in practicing meditation? Would it serve a positive purpose in their treatment plan? If so, is the client's ANS sufficiently balanced, and their mind calm enough, to benefit from an internally focused practice? Would they benefit from concentration exercises, such as gazing at a candle, to gain some mastery over the distractibility of their mind? Would an active meditation style, such as walking meditation, best serve the client? Or a passive style, such as nada yoga?)

_____

Successful NITYA-based therapy rests on an attitude of shared curiosity and exploration of the client's embodied experience. If a therapist shows an obvious interest and enthusiasm in hearing about their client's experience of the breath, for example, the client may feel supported enough to explore their breathing pattern. This exploration could organically lead to a memory, insight, or physiological shift. Even if it doesn't, the client may experience how their breathing pattern is intimately connected to their mood and ANS state. For example, a client, Lois, feels fearful every time she takes a breath. Rather than searching for the reasons why she might be fearful, which may elicit her cognitions, the skilled NITYA practitioner could begin by observing the client's natural breathing pattern and asking about any observable shifts. As the session continues, Lois may recognize that when she is thinking about something disturbing, her breath is shallow. This is accompanied by some anxiety in her chest. As she is coached by the therapist to deepen her breath, she suddenly feels more comfortable with the therapist, and sees the image of a smiley face. This intervention keeps the focus on her embodied present moment experience, which is all we really have to work with to diminish physiological trauma symptoms.

Yoga can be effective in whatever stage of healing the client is experiencing. While at first it may be a lifeline to sanity, it can become a health and mood enhancer. Finally, for some, it can become an ongoing experience of personal integration, complementing the gains made in psychotherapy. According to researcher Crystal L. Park, "The practice of yoga offers far more than physical postures and headstands – there is self-reflection, the practice of kindness and compassion, and continued growth and awareness" (Park et al., 2016).

Preparing to do this work: the therapist's embodiment and self-care

You can assess your degree of embodiment by examining your relationship with your body.

Does it require special attention, or does it just hum along to the tune of the habits you have already established? If you experience somatic distress, do you pay attention to it, and give yourself the time and resources, such as exercise, creative movement, yoga or massage, to address it? If not, what is getting in your way? If you struggle to find the motivation, or time, to address your somatic issues, would you consider going to a somatically-oriented professional for help?

In this model, the most important trait of the therapist/instructor, and one which may take time to develop, is an ability to maintain a state of ANS regulation in the face of the dysregulated nervous system state of the client. To prepare for working with NITYA, I encourage the therapist to undergo the same assessment they use with the client and practice the NITYA yoga techniques. The therapist self-assessment can include asking:

- Do you have any medical condition, or are you taking any medication, which should be taken into consideration when creating your NITYA-influenced plan?

- Of the four dimensions of health (physical, mental, emotional, and energetic/spiritual), which is the strongest in you? Which is most underdeveloped?

- What is the overall pattern of your defense cascade?

- What is your analysis of the current state of regulation of your own ANS?

- What are the symptoms which alert you to your dysregulation?

- Which interventions most effectively address your symptoms? Please be as specific as possible:

  Moral/ethical practices.

Physical interventions.

Breathing practices.

Deep relaxation/yoga nidra.

Meditation.

A case example

This example contains many of the elements which I have been describing in this book. It includes the influence of implicit memories on current behavior, as evidenced by the client's somatic issues. It the uses the assessment tool to note the client's medical history; explain the state of her ANS; identify the stage of her defense cascade, and of the corresponding gunas; and focus on inner resources. It recognizes the importance of safety to her progress; and encourages an awareness of body sensations in a bottom-up intervention. It uses a titrated approach to the recounting of her history.

Techniques used include the gradual introduction of chair yoga poses; psychoeducation about the connection between movement and trauma release; and an exploration of the relationship between the breathing pattern and feelings of aliveness. It also acknowledges the role that cognitively-based, top-down interventions can play; emphasizes the value of orientation to the external environment; and facilitates the client's experience of her own subtle energy.

Kate is a 22-year-old woman who was occasionally physically abused by her father when she was a child. She was terrified when he took his belt off to hit her, which he did on occasion. At those moments, she was not offered much support by other family members, so she ran off by herself to cry and try to comfort herself. She reports that she was able to do this to some degree, but also lost some connection to her deepest feelings and sensations, which, generally, left her chronically uncomfortable around men.

When she started dating in college, she felt "frozen" for the first half of the evening, unable to feel her body sensations, take a deep breath, or be at ease. Unable to explain this state to her dates, she was not asked out again. Kate reports chronic tension in her upper back and neck, which contributes to headaches, further limiting her ability to relax and express herself. The tension is particularly severe during holiday periods, when she is barely able to function.

When discomfort turned to despair, Kate decided to begin therapy with a psychotherapist/yoga instructor, Sue, with training in a nervous system-informed, trauma-sensitive approach, as well as other treatment modalities.

Chapter 6

Sue evaluated Kate using the NITYA assessment form. She began by asking Kate whether she was open to using movement and messages from her body, which she agreed to. (If not, I would recommend discontinuing this approach.) Sue then asked her if she had any chronic medical conditions, which she didn't. Through observation and inquiries, Sue determined that Kate's current ANS state was chronic tonic immobility. Clues to Kate's state were her lack of connection with her embodied experience, her low energy, her inability to express her discomfort, and her tendency toward shallow breathing.

On the positive side, Sue also noted Kate's willingness to learn, good physical health, and areas in her life of normal functioning. Sue believed that, gradually, Kate could make the shift from immobility, to freeze, to fight-or-flight, and continue to move up the defense cascade, to normal functioning. Sue explained the NITYA model to Kate, so that she would understand what was happening in her body, and could cooperate more fully in the process.

From that assessment, the therapist created a yoga-based treatment plan. This was part of a larger therapeutic plan, which included another well-known psychotherapeutic approach. (See the charts on ANS regulation using hatha yoga and breathing practices, discussed in Chapters 2 and 3.)

In the sessions, Sue first described the NITYA model which supported the interventions to Kate. She then introduced grounding exercises, such as feeling the connection between the back of the body and the chair, and noticing the natural flow of the breath, When Kate seemed to be slipping deeper into immobility, Sue introduced yoga postures geared to Kate's nervous system state, which Kate was able to do. When, later in therapy, Kate did begin to emerge into fight-or-flight, and her arm and leg muscles began to tense, the therapist assured her that this shift, while feeling uncomfortable, was a sign of progress toward ANS regulation. At this point, Kate spontaneously began to breathe more deeply, and the yogic three-part breath, performed with the exhale longer than the inhale, became a valuable nervous system-regulating tool.

Sue sometimes led Kate in the first section of yoga nidra, the progressive deep relaxation, which intensified, and then released, muscular tension. At moments when Kate's ANS was regulated, she reported feeling more energetic and content than she could ever remember feeling. Because she was able to be more present, she made significant progress using the other treatment modality.

The yoga treatment plan included a recording made by the therapist of a regular home practice of a sequence of chair yoga postures, executed at a moderate pace. The purpose of postures was to deepen Kate's connection with her body sensations; help her maintain her general health and flexibility; and when she felt anxious, downregulate her SNS by emphasizing forward bends. It also included the three-part deep breath, practiced for the first few minutes with an equal inhale and exhale, then shifting to a pattern with an exhale twice as long as the inhale, to encourage more SNS downregulation. In addition to this regular

practice, the client was encouraged to use mini-yoga interventions, such as a single posture or a few deep breaths, on her own, each time she started to feel more dysregulated.

In the next section of the book, we will look at the more subtle practices of yoga nidra and meditation as embodied tools for recovering from trauma.

Nervous system-informed, trauma-sensitive yoga nidra

Ellen had been in psychotherapy for five years with a trauma therapist whom she deeply trusted. She had made great progress in healing her early trauma, but was having difficulty sleeping. At one point, her therapist asked her if she would like to try a relaxation practice from the yoga tradition called yoga nidra. Ellen said yes, and, over the course of 10 sessions, carefully observing her and titrating the experience, the therapist led her through practice one stage at a time. After each stage, the therapist checked in with Ellen about her experience, and observed her ANS state, before proceeding to the next one. It was a testament to the resilience of Ellen's autonomic nervous system that she was able to experience all of the stages of NITYA yoga nidra without becoming dysregulated. Ellen enjoyed this experience, where she felt like she was hovering between sleep and wakefulness. When the experience was over, she felt deeply peaceful.

Pratyahara and sense withdrawal

Pratyahara, the Sanskrit term for "sense withdrawal," is the fifth branch of the Raja Yoga tree. In sense withdrawal, the experiencer gradually withdraws their attention, and energy, from a connection with the outer world of the senses, with its constant stimulation, to their inner experience. This is a major step toward the state of absorption which characterizes deep meditation. (There is empirical evidence that, in the context of meditation, a practice closely related to yoga nidra, sense withdrawal reduces brain activity and optimizes a feeling of inner peace through the reduction in incoming sensory stimuli (Newberg et al., 2000; 2002; 2010).)

Its principal practice is yoga nidra, the "yogic sleep," which is commonly defined as a state where the mind is awake while the body is asleep. This chapter provides an overview of the elements which comprise the practice; clarifies the NITYA perspective; and offers guidance to yoga therapists and mental health professionals who want to incorporate it into their work.

Yoga nidra basics

The practice of yoga nidra developed from general guidelines laid out in texts, which refer to the state without describing the process of achieving it. These texts include the Yoga Sutras of Patañjali (Sutra I.10), the Hatha Yoga Pradipika (Verse IV.43–50), the Mandukya Upanishad, and the Yoga Taravali, among others (Rama, 1982; Patañjali, 2003). This lack of specificity has led to the development of many styles of yoga nidra.

Current yoga nidra practices range from the nurturing experience of resting in a safe space while being sung to, as developed by Uma Dinsmore-Tuli in Total Yoga Nidra, to the highly-structured, researched, clinical model of cognitive, emotional, and sensory integration of iRest, with many variations in between. The NITYA approach is based on the Integral Yoga® model of yoga nidra, adapted for trauma-sensitivity.

I describe the NITYA approach to yoga nidra as a structured experience which is designed to progressively release muscle tension, regulate the ANS, reduce emotional charge, quiet cognitive activity, if and when the nervous system is regulated and the practitioner is ready, to shift the experience from body awareness into an experience of more subtle states.

This is a very significant shift for the trauma survivor. In the model of yoga nidra which I am presenting, the practice is a bridge between an embodied experience and an energetic one. As the guide across the bridge, the therapist must know the client well enough, and observe them closely enough, to be able to provide sufficient structure to ensure that the client will not fall into the abyss. That may mean traveling part way, gaining the benefits, and turning back.

The therapeutic application of yoga nidra

The therapeutic, trauma-sensitive practice of yoga nidra is primarily an embodied, bottom-up practice, done with the goal of calming a pattern of SNS overarousal. The practice can provide some clients some relief from muscle tension, racing thoughts, and other symptoms of SNS overactivation, and offer an experience of deep rest, which is a rare state not only for trauma survivors, but for many people living in the current, fast-paced world. On the physical level, this may be the result of increased dopamine release, found experimentally to be a result of yoga nidra practice (Kjaer et al., 2002).

For clients who are regulated enough to stay present to their internal experience, the internal focus generated by yoga nidra can be therapeutically valuable because, according to the Yoga Sutras, Sutra II.8, a preoccupation with external gratification is one of the factors that can perpetuate mental disorders (Satchidānanda, 1978, p. 106). One of the goals of yoga is to remove, or at least reduce, these preoccupations and

replace them with the experience of inner peace (Vahia et al., 1973.)

Two structures which support yoga nidra

Two frameworks which I believe underlie various approaches to yoga nidra are the brain wave model, based on contemporary science, and the kosha model, based on ancient teachings.

Yoga nidra and brain wave states

(NOTE: Unfortunately, the research that could definitively scientifically validate the following information has, to my knowledge, not yet been published. These theories are based on two unpublished laboratory experiments and the experience of highly developed yoga practitioners.)

One way I describe yoga nidra practice is as a journey through brain waves states, from the active, externally-oriented states, to the slower, internally-oriented ones (Mangalteertham, 1998). In everyday life, the brain produces beta brain waves, moving at 14–100 cycles per second. In this state, the mind is busy thinking and reacting. The practice of yoga nidra may initially put the practitioner in an alpha wave state (Desai, 2017, p. 38). Alpha brainwaves are slower than beta, moving at between nine and 14 cycles/second, and produce a state of relaxed wakefulness (Desai, 2017, p. 39). As the practice deepens, theta and delta wave states may begin to predominate. The frequency of theta is 5–8 cycles/second. It is a dreamy state, where the individual can experience a progression of images and thoughts without being affected by them, as if they were watching a movie (Desai, 2017, pp. 40–41). Delta waves, present in deep, dreamless sleep, are slower still, at 1.5 to 4 cycles/

second (Herrmann, 1997). These frequencies bring the individual almost to the point of the cessation of brain waves, which is similar to the definition of yoga in the Yoga Sutras, described in Chapter 1. In that state, the body can deeply rest and a person can experience inner peace, which is considered in the yogic tradition to be our true nature (Satchidananda, 2011; Kesarcodi-Watson, 1982.) These states correspond to the dissolution of the sense of "I" for the experiencer, along with a complete loss of body awareness (Desai, 2017, p. 50), and are similar to those described by Swami Veda Bharati in his writings about yoga nidra (Bharati, 2014).

The experience of yoga nidra as a spiritual practice has been defined as the ability to remain fully conscious while in the delta wave state, characteristic of deep sleep (Parker et al., 2013, p. 11). Swami Rama, founder of the Pennsylvania-based Himalayan Institute, demonstrated this phenomenon in 1970, at the Menninger Clinic. He participated in an EEG study of yoga nidra in a laboratory setting, where he was observed entering yoga nidra for about 10 minutes, during which time delta waves were recorded. He was then able to repeat verbatim all the conversations that had occurred in the lab during that time (Green & Green, 1977).

An accidental experiment with Swami Veda Bharati, internationally known Vedic scholar and student of Swami Rama, produced similar results. While the Swami was carrying on a conversation with Dean Radin, PhD., at the Institute for Noetic Sciences, in preparation for a yoga nidra experiment, Dr. Radin noticed that the leads were attached to the Swami, and the EEG recorder was running. It showed that the Swami was producing mainly delta waves in his normal "waking state" (Bharati, 2006, p. 69).

Yoga nidra and the kosha model

According to traditional texts, when withdrawing the senses, the practitioner can gain greater access to energy sheaths which surround the body, called "koshas," than in waking normal consciousness (Figure 7.1). The kosha model was introduced in the second chapter of Taittirīya Upanishad, the Ananda Valli, a Vedic-era Sanskrit text most likely composed in, or close to, the 6th century BC (Shankaracharya & Angot, 2007). Access to these sheaths can bring greater awareness to the individual of their current physical condition, energy state, thought patterns, and intuition (Ashok & Thimmappa, 2006). Bringing this awareness into daily life can help to transform that experience, even if external day-to-day conditions remain the same.

These sheaths are said to be connected to the physical body in layers, moving from gross to

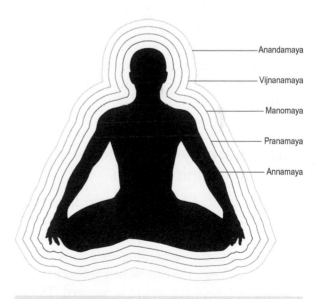

- Anandamaya
- Vijnanamaya
- Manomaya
- Pranamaya
- Annamaya

FIGURE 7.1 The koshas.

subtle. According to Swami Satyananda, on reaching the most subtle level, practitioners can transform their deepest psychological conditioning (Saraswati & Hiti, 1984). (To my knowledge, this assertion is as yet scientifically unproven, though some anecdotal evidence does exist.)

The grossest sheath, which is the most tightly tied to sensual awareness, is the annamaya kosha, the physical body, which translates as the "food body." The next sheath is the pranamaya kosha, the domain of the subtle nerves and the prana which infuses them. The third sheath, the manomaya kosha, contains our thoughts. The next sheath, vijnanamaya kosha, which translates as "composed of special knowledge," connects us to our intuition. Anandamaya kosha, the fifth sheath, means "bliss body." Swami Satyananda describes this sheath as a storehouse of impressions from the past and the key to transforming our personality. The progression of the koshas recapitulates the potential for spiritual development described in the practices of Raja Yoga, from hatha yoga for the body; to pranayama for the breath; to sense withdrawal, to gain access to deep inner experience; and to the mental deconditioning found in meditation.

Yoga nidra, polyvagal theory, and related clinical issues

Up to this point, I have emphasized the moral and ethical principles, postures, and breathing practices which strengthen ANS regulation. With yoga nidra, and the succeeding meditative disciplines of Raja Yoga, the connection between these practices and ANS regulation is reversed. These passive experiences, which lack volitional movement and significant SNS involvement, can either activate the ventral/dorsal hybrid state, or invite the unconscious process of neuroception, which involves scanning for danger. This is a defensive response which is not conducive to surrender, which is the quality necessary to experience the subtlety of the practices. Therefore, significant periods of stillness in the practice are not recommended for trauma survivors who are struggling to achieve a ventral/dorsal state (Porges, 2017).

In addition, as the yoga practitioner advances in yoga nidra practices, the physiological supports, mediated by the cranial nerves and described by polyvagal theory as promoting ANS regulation, are gradually removed. These include: first, social engagement, as the yoga nidra practitioner withdraws from relationships with others, to focus on internal experiences; then movement, as I have just mentioned, since the instruction is to remain still. Loss of movement is followed by the loss of visual contact with the external environment, in that the eyes generally close as the individual deepens their practice; then vocalization, as silence is maintained; and, in its last stage, hearing, since the yoga nidra instructor maintains silence for an extended period of time. These factors comprise a discipline which goes beyond the senses, and emphasizes the internal independence of the experiencer, which rests on their inherent ANS regulation, rather than their capacity for social engagement.

On the surface, it seems that the later stages of yoga nidra would not be appropriate for trauma survivors, and this is a widespread belief held by yoga therapy professionals. However, an analysis of the practice I am familiar with, and am presenting in this chapter, raises deeper questions about issues in working with trauma survivors, and even how the term is defined.

As Dr. Schwartz writes in the Foreword, "most people will experience at least one traumatic event in their lifetime and … exposure to multiple traumatic events is the norm" (Kilpatrick at al., 2013). That research expands the population of individuals at risk for destabilizing triggers, to the majority. And, in the case of trauma, a diagnosis may not provide sufficient information upon which to make a clinical decision concerning the selection of yoga practices. An email exchange between myself and Dr. Porges highlighted the complexity of this issue. He wrote: "From my perspective … categorizing trauma survivors as a 'group' is problematic, since it focuses on the trauma event and not the experience. Thus, yogic and meditative practices may have embedded triggers linked to shifts in autonomic state for some survivors and not others" (Porges, private correspondence, February 10, 2021).

The upshot of this discussion is that I urge therapists to learn as much as possible about their client's inner world; be as attentive as possible to the client's state shifts; become very familiar with the practices which they are using with clients through their own experience; establish as strong a relationship with the client as possible; be cautious in the use of the more internal practices; and, at the same time, leave an opening for an exploration of deeper territory, after obtaining the client's consent. I am presenting four stages of yoga nidra practice with the hope that they offer enough choices to provide safety to clients at various levels of regulation.

The NITYA style of yoga nidra

NITYA Yoga Nidra is based on Integral Yoga® Nidra, developed by Swami Satchidananda.

This original formulation consists of four phases, based on the koshas, moving from an experience of embodiment to one of internal energetic absorption. The deepening of the practice correlates with the step-by-step release of body consciousness. These phases make this version trauma-sensitive, since they gradually shift the focus from the body, to the breath, to the thoughts, and finally to a quiet, peaceful place beyond the thoughts, in distinct segments. They can be used as touchstones for progress in trauma healing. As I indicate in the script, an exploration of the first phase is safe with most clients. Before going on to the other phases, optimally, a client should be able to comfortably complete a trauma-sensitive yoga chair or mat sequence, and breathing practices. It is most beneficial to instruct the client in a complete sequence of both just before starting the yoga nidra, as a tune-up for their ANS.

Phase one

In NITYA, the practitioner begins at the body level, the annamaya kosha, with the progressive deep relaxation, the tensing and relaxing of the major muscle groups. The guided relaxation decreases muscular tension and provides access to a wider range of sensations (Coulter, 2012, p. 561). This practice alternately stimulates the SNS and PNS, encouraging their healthy oscillation (Johnson, 2009). I am aware of a controversy in the use of the word "relaxation" in the teaching of yoga nidra and other relaxation techniques. On one side of the issue, the word sounds like a directive to some trauma survivors which they may not want, or be able, to follow. In a more mindful approach, the individual would be directed to notice the sensations which are present. On the other side there is a physiological benefit to the act of tensing and then releasing, the muscles.

Chapter 7

I have used the word "relaxation" in my yoga nidra script, and suggest that it can be changed to "be aware of" a muscle or body part for individuals who feel more comfortable with that term.

The client can also be encouraged to reduce the activity of the cranial nerves through resting the eyes; releasing muscles of the nose; allowing the tongue to soften; releasing the muscles associated with the ears; and letting the skin on the face soften. (See the discussion of the action of the cranial nerves in Chapter 1.)

Phase one of the NITYA model is designed to be ANS-balancing and is safe for most clients. I associate this phase of yoga nidra with the transition from beta to alpha brain waves, producing relaxed alertness.

Phase two

This section of the practice is most suitable for individuals who were able to successfully practice phase one and are able to feel safe, in a hybrid ventral/dorsal vagal state, without moving. In this phase, the client mindfully focuses on the areas they relaxed in the previous phase, beginning with the feet and moving to the scalp, mentally sending additional messages of release. This is the beginning of a process of disidentification from the body, which is a peaceful experience for some people, and, in my experience, of transitioning from alpha to theta brain wave states.

Phase three

In phase three, which is closely related but requires more ANS regulation, the client is instructed to visualize healing energy slowly spreading from the scalp, down the body. While the point of reference is still the body, it is experienced in a more diffuse way, with the assistance of visualization. When successfully completing phase three, the participant may experience the transition from an alpha brain wave state to a dreamy theta state.

Phase four

Phase four is an advanced practice appropriate for the small percentage of clients who can remain regulated when in a hybrid ventral/dorsal state, when their awareness is drawn inward and body awareness is minimized. This is because the unstructured, open nature of this phase gives latitude for the troubled mind to wander back to overwhelming fears and traumatic memories. In this phase, the client is instructed to observe their natural breathing pattern for one minute; observe their thoughts for one minute; then dwell in a state that is deeper than the thoughts for up to five minutes, in silence. They are instructed to come out of the practice if they begin to feel any discomfort.

This is a powerful progression. Breath observation can engage the pranamaya kosha and can produce a feeling of calm in the body and mind. Observing the thoughts without identifying with them can help the practitioner to detach from the activity of their manomaya kosha, and therefore remain less affected by its contents. For the unusual client who feels safe being with their inner experience, during the up to five-minute period of silence, as mental activity ceases, they may be unaware of the passage of time; may feel like a force greater than themself is breathing them; and may lose body awareness. In this stage, in NITYA theory, the practitioner may be hovering between the theta wave state and the delta state of deep sleep, but with full awareness of each moment. In this state, the individual can choose to disidentify with the body and its tensions, pain, illnesses, and patterns from the past; with the mind, with its incessant, charged thoughts; and with a limiting, socially constructed self-concept, dependent upon external validation. Ideally, in returning from this inner journey, former self-identifications can be loosened, and at least partially replaced, with a connection to an experience of innate peace and joy, independent of mental programming and external circumstances. This state is called turiya in the yoga tradition, the state beyond being awake, sleeping, or dreaming (Birch & Hargreaves, 2015). Yoga nidra can be an experience of the yogic teaching that we are essentially not our body or our mind but, rather, an energetic essence (Miller, 2012). This shift in identification is, traditionally, a major feature of spiritual development and a foundation for understanding yoga nidra, and spiritually-oriented yoga practices in general. Completing phase four is a milestone in trauma resolution, and the fulfillment of the promise of yoga nidra for those who are ready.

In this four-phase adaptation for the trauma survivor, the therapist and client can decide together how far to go in the process, based on the client's goals and state of regulation. If, during the practice, any defensive responses, disturbing memories, images, or emotions are evoked for the client, I suggest ending the practice there, re-establishing safety, and noticing any benefits which may have accrued. I recommend this not only because of the possibility of dissociation, which can result in retraumatization, but also because the practice would not yield benefits for the client if they are experiencing emotional or physical dis-ease.

SCRIPT

Annotated script for trauma-sensitive yoga nidra

Adapted from the Integral Yoga® Hatha Teacher Training manual ©2017 Satchidananda Ashram–Yogaville Inc. Used with permission. See Appendix 5 for the script without notes.

Part one: progressive deep relaxation *(for all clients)*

I am going to lead you through yoga nidra, the yogic sleep, into a state of deep relaxation. You can sit or lie down, and have your eyes open or closed, whatever is more comfortable for you. Feel free to interrupt me at any time if you have a question or problem by raising your hand, and please discontinue the practice at any time if you feel uncomfortable.

(Speaking slowly.) You are invited to notice the points of contact between the back of your body and surface you are relaxing on. (Pause.) Tune into the natural flow of your breath. (Pause.) Now, bring your awareness to your right foot and leg. Stretch out the toes, then tense the muscles of the foot and leg. *(Increase the intensity of your voice.)* Raise it a few inches off the floor, hold, squeeze, then let it gently fall back to the floor. Roll the leg from side to side and let it go. (Pause.) Focus on the breath for two breaths.

Now stretch out the toes of your left foot. *(Increase the intensity of your voice.)* Tense the muscles of the foot and leg. Raise it a few inches off of the floor … holding, tightening … then release it. Roll it from side to side and let it go. (Pause.) Again, focus on the breath.

Focusing on your right hand, stretch out the fingers, then make a fist. *(Increase the intensity of your voice.)* Tense the muscles of the right hand and arm and raise it a few inches. Hold … tense … relax, and release. Roll it from side to side, and let it go. (Pause.) Notice the breath.

Focusing on your left hand, stretch out the fingers, then make a fist. *(Increase the intensity of your voice.)* Continue by tensing it, raising, and holding. Release the arm, rolling it from side to side, and let it go. (Pause.) Focus on the breath for two breaths.

Focusing on the buttock muscles, the ones you sit on, squeeze them together. *(Increase the intensity of your voice.)* Hold, tighten, and let them go. Roll the hips gently from side to side. (Pause.)

Focus on the breath. After your next exhalation, inhale deeply through the nose, into the abdomen, blowing it up like a balloon. *(Increase the intensity of your voice.)* Take in a little more air, a little more, and, through an open mouth, release it! Now, inhale into the chest, filling the chest with air. *(Increase the intensity of your voice.)* Take in a little more air, a little more, then, through an open mouth, release it! Let the breath return to normal and watch it for three breaths. (Pause.)

Bring your awareness to your shoulders. First, as you exhale, squeeze the shoulders together toward the center of the chest. Hold, squeeze, and release. Then, as you inhale, compress the shoulder blades toward the center of the back, feeling the chest expand and the back arching. Release the shoulders as you exhale. (Pause.) Now, as you inhale, raise the shoulders, as if to touch the ears. Squeeze, and release. Then, exhaling, press them down toward the feet, and release them. Gently roll the head from side to side, as you watch the breath. (Pause.)

Open your mouth and roll the jaw around. (Pause.) Now close your mouth and, as you inhale, suck in the cheeks, and pucker the lips. Exhale, and release. (Pause.) As you inhale, tense the muscles of the nostrils, and release with an exhalation. Inhale, knitting the eyebrows together in the center of your forehead; exhale and release. Inhale again, raising the eyebrows toward the top of the head. Exhale and release. (Pause.) Take a breath.

Now, as you inhale, make your face as long as you can by opening your mouth, sticking out your tongue, pointing it toward your feet, and looking up toward the top of your head. Release. Now do just the opposite: inhale as you bring all of the facial features together into a ball in the center of the face. Squeeze … and release. Do that one more time, and release. Again, gently roll the head from side to side, and bring it back to center. Please take a breath. (Pause.)

Part two: body scan *(for clients who are comfortable with, and are able to do, a mental scan of their body parts while continuing to breathe)*

Now that you have relaxed the major muscles of the body, you can use the power of suggestion, the power of the mind, to relax the body a little bit more. Without moving, except for the flow of the breath, bring your awareness to your toes, (pause) soles of the feet, (pause) and tops of the feet, (pause), sending them a mental suggestion to release a little bit more. (Brief pause after each body part named.) Release the lower legs, knees, upper legs, buttocks muscles, and finally the entire pelvis. Please take a breath. (Pause.)

Bring your awareness to your hands. (Brief pause after each body part named.) Release muscular tension in the fingers, palms, back of the hands, lower arms, elbows, upper arms, and shoulders. (Pause.) Take a breath. Now, bring your awareness to the abdominal area. Release muscular tension in the abdominal organs, ribcage, lungs, and chest. Please take a breath. (Pause.)

(Brief pause after each body part named.) Bring your awareness to your back. Release tension in the lower back, middle back, and upper back, feeling every point of contact between your back and surface you are resting on. (Pause.)

(Brief pause after each body part named.) Relax the throat, jaw, cheeks, lips, teeth, and even the tongue. Relax the nose, eyes, eyebrows, forehead, and scalp. Please take a breath. (Pause.)

Part three: visualizing peaceful energy
(for clients with good body awareness who can lie still for a few minutes, and are comfortable with a visualization exercise)

(Speak slowly and softly.) Feel that your scalp is being bathed in a peaceful energy which is slowly spreading down the torso, arms, and legs, revitalizing and rejuvenating every cell (one minute of complete silence).

Part four: silent witnessing *(for clients experienced in yoga and who feel confident in regulating their own nervous system, who are not consciously engaging in injurious behavior toward themselves or others)*

Now bring your awareness to your breath. Watch the breath as it flows in and out. Don't try to control it; just watch. Be a silent witness to the flow of the breath. (Pause for 30 seconds.) Continue to watch the breath. (30 seconds of complete silence.)

Now shift your awareness to your thoughts. Don't be attached to them, just watch them, as if you were watching a movie. (Pause for 30 seconds.) Continue to watch the thoughts. (30 seconds of complete silence.)

Now see if you can find a place that is deeper than the thoughts, a place where there are no thoughts. If you find this peaceful place, just enjoy it. If not, you can watch the thoughts, or watch the breath. (Up to 5 minutes of silence.) Please let me know if you start to feel uncomfortable.

Bring your awareness back to your breath, deepening it. (Pause.) Start to wake the body by moving the fingers and toes, arms, and legs. When you are ready, you can open your eyes, roll onto your right side, and slowly sit up. (Pause.) Now look around the room, letting your eyes go where they want to go, until they come back to a centered gaze. This is the end of the yoga nidra practice.

Yoga nidra in the session

Following trauma-sensitive yoga guidelines described in Chapter 2, the physical space where yoga nidra is performed should be comfortable, private, and quiet (Emerson et al., 2011). Participants should be offered as many practice options as possible, such as sitting or lying down, with the eyes open or closed. It would be helpful to offer the client a blanket, since the client's body may cool a few degrees as the skin releases heat, when the PNS becomes dominant (Coulter, 2012, p. 556).

If working with an individual in a private session, I recommend, first, determining the client's ability to self-regulate, since that determines which stage(s) of the practice are the most appropriate for that client. Then, the therapist can have a treatment goal in mind when offering this practice (as all interventions should), as yoga nidra can take up to 30 minutes out of valuable session time to administer.

For example, the therapist can assess the client for conditions which respond well to a gentle contraction and release of the muscles and calming of the ANS, such as chronic muscle tension, frequent headaches, chronic disease, insomnia, somatic symptom disorders, anxiety-related conditions, and many PTSD symptoms. Examples from my practice have included clients with multiple sclerosis and chronic pain, individuals struggling with anxiety, and those dealing with the side effects of withdrawal from anti-anxiety medication. If yoga nidra does not seem like the best intervention for a particular client, the therapist can use NITYA yoga postures and breathing practices instead to achieve their therapeutic goals.

The deeper the client goes into the practice, the more time it may take afterwards for them to emerge into everyday, beta-wave consciousness. When this practice is administered, I recommend leaving ample time in the session for reentering and grounding. It can be effective to engage the client's neo-cortex at the end the process, by asking cognitively stimulating questions.

I strongly recommend that the therapist who uses yoga nidra with clients has personally experienced the stages of practice, and can assess the level which is most appropriate for the client. Additionally, the peace and joy which the therapist may have experienced in the practice can often be communicated through tone of voice, posture, attitude, and energy. If the client would benefit from practicing yoga nidra at home, I recommend the creation of an individually-tailored recording for home practice.

Caution

> When the mind has transcended maya [illusion] when the ego has become static, when senses are no longer functioning, and when all communication of the mind and the senses has been cut, when you and I no longer exist for a period of time, yoga nidra starts.
>
> Sri Shakaracharya,
> Yoga Taravalli (8th century CE)

Yoga nidra taught without trauma sensitivity is a wild card which may be dangerous for the client. At one extreme, many years ago, a student in one of my neighborhood wellness classes, who was not aware of previous trauma in her life, sat up in the middle of my yoga nidra instruction and ran out of the room, then the building. She later told me that she had been gripped with an unexplained feeling of terror. At the other extreme, I met a man at a human potential center who had had a history of intense anxiety for approximately 30 years.

He had tried many approaches to heal it, to no avail. Five years prior to our meeting, he had taken a weekend yoga nidra workshop with a well-known yoga master from India. After this first yoga nidra experience, when he opened his eyes, the anxiety was gone, and it had not returned. He was taking that yoga nidra program again, in celebration.

Even with the safeguards built into the titration of the process, yoga nidra may still trigger uncomfortable memories and/or body sensations which may take the experiencer by surprise.

I recommend co-creating and practicing simple protocols with the client which can alert the therapist to stop the process, such as raising their hand, making a sound, or calling for help.

Yoga nidra is a structured experience which is designed to progressively release muscle tension, regulate the ANS, reduce emotional charge, quiet cognitive activity, and shift the experience from body awareness into an experience of more subtle states. It has much in common with meditation, which will be explored in the next chapter.

Betty is well into her trauma recovery process when she walks into the meditation room for a 20-minute period of silent meditation. In this safe environment, having prepared herself by developing a flexible body, focused mind, and strong motivation, Betty is usually able to sit still and focus on her breath and body sensations. However, during practice today, as the minutes go by, she begins to feel tension in the pit of her stomach which distracts her from the practice to such a degree that she needs to stop. She decides to do a walking meditation instead, which allows her to discharge some of that tension and bring her back into ANS regulation.

The term "meditation" is a catch-all phrase, since there are different forms, from various traditions, practiced at varying levels of intensity. But essentially, they have one thing in common: they all train the individual to simultaneously experience the thoughts in their conditioned mind, and the silence of pure awareness. Some traditions include body sensations as a meditative focus. In this chapter, I am offering an overview of a few of these practices, which include the embodied meditation techniques of walking meditation and nada yoga, the yoga of sound, which I see as trauma sensitive.

Traditional styles of yogic meditation

Before we explore other styles of meditation, I want to describe the Raja Yoga form of meditation (termed "dhyana" in Sanskrit), which is limb number seven of the eight-limbed path (Figure 8.1). In this system, meditation it is the culmination of a long process (Satchidananda, 1978). The goal of the practice is to quiet mental activity (Sivananda, 2009). The preparation involves cultivating an ethical lifestyle with the yamas and niyamas (ethical precepts), so the individual avoids creating inner disturbances; performing simple yoga postures, whereby the individual strengthens their body for extended periods of sitting; directing the flow of prana with breathing exercises, so that the individual masters the mental restlessness; developing the ability to rest peacefully in one's inner world (pratyahara); and strengthening the capacity to focus attention (dharana), before moving on to meditation.

8 Samhadi
Bliss which defies description

7 Dhyana
Meditation

Contemplation

Meditation

Concentration

6 Dharana
Steadying the mind

5 Pratyahara
Sense withdrawal

Controls of sense

4 Pranayama
Breathing technique

Control of breath/life force

3 Asana
Posture and movement

Control of body

Purity

Contentment

Austerity

Self study

2 Niyama
Things to do, coming to terms with yourself

Truthfulness

Non injury

Dedication

1 Yama
Self restraints

Non theft

Spiritual conduct

Non greed

Discipline

Self study

Dedication

Figure 8.1 Raja Yoga tree.

This style of meditation is done sitting in an erect posture, as motionless as possible, for an extended period of time. The meditator sits with the eyes half-opened, or closed, silently focusing on a sound, the breath, or on the thoughts. This practice can have great benefits for the resilient practitioner. For this individual, the structure of the practice, the protected quality of the meditation space, and the lack of external stimulation, all provide the ideal situation to turn their awareness inward, to depths uncharted by polyvagal theory. However, I do not recommend it for most trauma survivors in early to mid-stages of recovery. This practice provides a counterpoint to the brain's natural state, called the "default mode network." This is because it is too unstructured, leaving open the possibility of reverting to the default mode network. This network is active during resting wakefulness, where one has the tendency to daydream. This type of activity can lead the trauma survivor into thought patterns which are retraumatizing (Alves et al., 2019).

There are two basic forms of seated yogic meditation: focused and open (also called "nondirective"). Focused meditation traditionally uses the rhythm of the breath, or the silent repetition of a Sanskrit syllable or phrase, or "mantra," as the focus. While this technique would invite dissociation in some trauma survivors, it may be a valuable tool to others by interrupting negative or obsessive thought patterns. In traditional yoga practice, the mantra is more than a tool to focus the mind; it claims that the sound itself will eventually dissolve the mental patterns. According to Swami Sivananda, "Chanting of Mantras generates potent ... waves or ... vibrations. They penetrate the physical and ... [subtle] bodies of the patients and remove the root-causes of the sufferings..." (Sivananda,

2020a). (NOTE: This belief is no doubt foreign to Western minds, but it is an important basis for traditional yoga practice.)

In focused meditation, when the mind wanders, the practitioner is instructed to bring it back to the mantra and/or the breath, over and over again. This practice is an attempt to train the mind to be present and slowly wear away unconscious mind/body patterns which obscure, or distract from, present moment experience.

In an open style of yogic meditation, the goal is to experience each moment as fully as possible, with its passing thoughts, sensations, and emotions, without reacting to the experience. This process challenges chronic patterns of perception and belief. The open and focused styles can be combined, so that the client begins with the focused meditation and, once the mind is focused, continues with a more open style.

In either practice, by design, the stillness, silence, and extended inner focus can serve to weaken the natural barriers between the conscious and the unconscious mind, allowing the practitioner to more deeply experience the reactions which they know, and discover unconditioned inner states. This process clearly falls in the territory of yoga as a spiritual path, rather than a healing modality.

Looking at seated meditation from a polyvagal point of view, the result is similar to that in yoga nidra: the removal of most of the supports which help to regulate the ANS. If the individual experiences inner or outer threat, with the eyes either closed or open but unfocused, in a silent environment, social engagement and orienting for safety are not available. Without movement, there is no opening to fight or run away, so the only option is immobilization, which can deaden the practitioner to their experience, and/or inadvertently reopen avenues of unhealed trauma. On the other hand, for some individuals on the healing path with a regulated ANS, an open style of meditation, supported by the stillness and silence, can be a door to observation of the subtle, reciprocal interplay between thoughts, images, and the ANS responses, which can open to greater self-knowledge.

Meditation as cognitive therapy

Meditation contains a cognitive element and can be a useful cognitive therapy tool. The Yoga Sutras mention a specific technique, pratipaksha bhavana, or "thought substitution" (Sutra II.33–34), the practice of overcoming negative ways of thinking, through the discipline of cultivating opposite, positive thoughts (Satchidananda, 1978). In my opinion, a modern variation of this practice is to insert a more accurate thought, rather than the opposite one, to break a distorted thought pattern. For example, the client who is upset but in no real danger may say, "I'm afraid I'm going to die." The opposite thought would be "I'm not afraid I'm going to die." A more accurate thought would be, "I'm not in any real danger ... I'm afraid of death, but I know I'll be OK." This practice can balance the mental polarities illustrated in the NITYA Healing Chart and bring them closer to the center of the "yoga zone."

Benefits and cautions of meditation

I see traditional meditation practice for trauma survivors, whether open or focused, as a double-edged sword. On the positive side, if the meditator generally feels physically and emotionally safe, a traditional meditation practice has many benefits. It can minimize external stimulation to the senses, which allows the ANS to shift into a more deeply parasympathetic state. This shift can increase levels of oxytocin and GABA, which produce feelings of wellbeing (Davidson et al., 2003.; Khattab et al., 2007). As I have mentioned, the practice can decrease the activity of the default mode network. (NOTE: Oxytocin is a hormone and a neurotransmitter that is involved in childbirth and breastfeeding. It is also associated with empathy, trust, sexual activity, and relationship-building. GABA is a neurotransmitter which relieves anxiety and improves mood.)

In a different vein, studies have confirmed improved psychological wellbeing and cognitive functioning following meditation, due to the activation of attention networks (Rubia, 2009). The meditative components of yoga were found to increase levels of growth factors in the brain, which helps support existing neurons, encourages neuroplasticity through the growth and differentiation of new neurons, and counteract the degenerative effects of inflammation (Huang & Reichardt, 2001).

On the sword's negative edge, meditation, particularly intensive practice, can amplify unhealthy tendencies which were already present, even in individuals without a mental health diagnosis. For example, in meditation, the mindful but anxious person may over-focus on each body sensation, wondering if it is a symptom of disease, and create more anxiety. The dissociated person may further dissociate, losing awareness of body sensations. The depressed person may become more lethargic. Even for someone who generally feels emotionally and physically well, a meditation technique which brings their awareness into the present moment may uncover the unconscious content which was blocking their ability to be present in the first place, and intensify defensive responses. The minds of some individuals can become so disturbed that the meditative process is more like drowning than holding on to a life preserver, which is how meditation techniques are sometimes described.

A NITYA approach to meditation

In a NITYA approach to meditation, particularly for the individual in the initial stages of trauma recovery, I recommend an embodied practice, personalized to accommodate each individual. Practices such as walking meditation and nada yoga, the chanting of, and listening to, uplifting sounds, though not well researched, show great potential to be healing for the trauma survivor, who can strengthen their connection to their body sensations while they develop greater resources for inner exploration.

As with the other practices, my recommendations are only guidelines. There are many shades of gray in the effects of meditation on trauma recovery. A practice which is retraumatizing to one individual may be harmless, or even beneficial, to another. For example, in a therapy session with an alcoholic, suicidal client of mine, diagnosed with post-traumatic stress disorder (PTSD), I mentioned that in meditation, the practitioner examines their thoughts, welcoming some and discarding others. In my opinion, this is a high-level skill. This client suddenly realized that she did not have to believe all of her thoughts, many of which were internalized from people who had negative intentions toward her. This realization was a turning point. As she sat and examined the veracity of her thoughts about herself, she recovered her self-esteem, and was able to slowly give up her self-destructive behaviors.

Walking meditation

Walking meditation is a simple practice where the meditator focuses on the experience of walking slowly and deliberately, in a measured rhythm, while being aware of body sensations, as well as thoughts, images, and emotions. The right/left alternation of limbs, in itself, can be regulating to the ANS. The contact between the soles of the feet and the floor can be grounding, and provide a point of focus for a mind with a tendency toward dissociation. The need to visually scan the environment as one walks is naturally orienting. Undischarged fight-and-flight energy can be downregulated as a result of the muscular-driven forward movement. The slowing of movement can allow a natural deepening of the breath, stimulating the ventral vagus nerve. This practice, then, supports the client in the healing process on a physiological level.

Walking meditation can be done informally, geared to the client's preferences, or formally, following a protocol, which is more appropriate for a group setting. One example of a protocol is an agreement to restrict one's field of vision to the back of the person walking in front of them, providing a focus for the mind. The client can be encouraged to take breaks at any time, by stopping, or stepping aside (if in a group), connecting with the therapist, or just relaxing their concentration. Walking meditation has the potential to expand the client's "yoga zone" as they become more regulated and comfortable with their moment-to-moment experience.

Nada yoga

Chanting, singing, or even passively listening to chants of Sanskrit mantras and prayers are part of the path of Nada yoga, the yoga of sound. These are powerful, safe meditation practices for individuals with nervous system dysregulation. They are meditative because they naturally support the focusing of the mind, the relaxation of the body, and the dropping away of chronic mental patterns. They are powerful because, according to the Sat-Cakra-Nirupana, one of the earliest texts on the nadis and chakras, the sound of the letters of the Sanskrit language each vibrate a specific part of the physical body, offering healing to the body and mind (Avalon, 1974).

From my experience, when one is chanting or singing, it is difficult to think about anything! The music can be a lure which can bring the experiencer effortlessly into the present moment. From a Western, scientific point of view, benefits can come from the activation of the PNS via the ventral vagus nerve, through the vibration of the moveable bones in the inner ear, and from the vocalization of sound, which can release tension in the larynx and stimulate the vagus nerve. From an Eastern, yogic perspective, they come from the healing effect of the sound vibrations on the cells of the body. Research studies have shown some positive effects from mantra repetition, and no negative ones (Berkovich-Ohana, 2015).

Research also supports claims by practitioners of a soothing effect of "Om" chants. In one study, limbic system activity, closely related to SNS activity, was reduced when Om was chanted. The control group chanted an "sss" sound, which had no effect (Gangadhar et al., 2011). In another study, the chanting of Om produced an increase in theta wave amplitude, producing a reduction in cortical arousal and promoting relaxation (Harne & Hiwale, 2018). While additional research needs to be performed to replicate these findings, they highlight a potential role for Om chanting in clinical practice.

In another study, each repetition of the Ave Maria prayer, as well as yoga mantra chants, spoken in their original language, brought the practitioner's breathing rate to approximately six repetitions/minute. This is the same rate as "coherent breathing," a Western version of the yogic three-part deep breath. Research has shown that coherent breathing is health-enhancing, and increases heart rate variability and the flexibility of the ANS (Elliott, 2005; Bernardi et al., 2001). This finding highlights the potential benefits of many styles of singing and sounding which slow the breath which are outside of religious and spiritual traditions (Bolger & Judson, 1984).

The inclusion of these trauma-sensitive meditation techniques completes the description of the NITYA model of care, offering a full spectrum of techniques for individuals with symptoms of nervous system dysregulation.

Summary

A few weeks before writing this chapter, during the COVID-19 crisis, I was asked to give a NITYA training to school social workers employed by the New York City Board of Health. I emphasized that, first, the therapist needs to know how to monitor their own ANS and have, and use, resources to keep their own ANS balanced. Then, the therapist needs to become familiar with the effects of the yogic interventions, through their own practice. They then need to recognize the client's ANS pattern of dysregulation to know which intervention to choose, when, and in what amount. Finally, they need to feel confident in teaching a somatic intervention.

I stressed that the therapist must also understand the requirements of embodied healing for the trauma survivor: to recognize the mechanism behind the ANS's cascade of survival defenses, ranging from SNS high activation, to PNS shutdown; to see how that polarized pattern underlies the emotional, intellectual, and energetic life of the individual; and to know how that pattern can slowly be transformed, with patience, attention, and the right tools, into the more stable territory of the yoga zone. This zone is characterized by a smooth oscillation of the autonomic nervous system; contentment; present moment awareness; and "sattva," a peaceful and balanced energy state.

Toward the end of the presentation, one of the participants asked me to give specific suggestions, in addition to the yogic techniques, for working with this population. I answered that the most important factor was to maximize the emotional and physical safety of the students. This is because the ANS's first priority is survival. When someone feels unsafe, or is unsafe, the temporary symptoms of dysregulation which emerge are protective. However, in the long run, they often are damaging to the body and to the client's ability to learn and grow from their experiences.

I then reviewed recommendations from Polyvagal Theory. These included being in the company of regulated people, who themselves felt safe. Their regulated state would be evidenced by their relaxed facial muscles, particularly around their eyes; their friendly facial expressions and body gestures; their rhythmic vocal pattern and the welcoming tone of their voice; their diaphragmatic breathing pattern, and general easeful demeanor. Other suggestions I gave were to eat moderate portions of fresh, whole foods; get regular exercise and exposure to sunlight; and spend time in natural environments. All of these suggestions facilitate the healthy flow of prana. My answer came hesitatingly, because I realized that it could be difficult for these inner-city youth, approximately 85% of whom are minorities, and 17% of whose families lived in poverty in 2018, to access these healthful resources (Official Website of the City of New York, 2019; New York City Council, 2019).

It is important, however, to state that these resources, while unavailable for many now, could be plentiful if our society valued every member, regardless of their race, ethnic group, gender, age, disability level, education and income level; if we truly prioritized their wellbeing, and were committed to implementing a model of healthcare which optimizes ANS balance and utilizes the insights which NITYA, and the yoga tradition, offer.

Afterword: Seeing the light

Peace is the most important factor in growth and development. It is in the tranquility of the night that the seed slowly sprouts from under the soil. The bud opens in the depth of the most silent hours. So also, in a state of peace and love, people evolve, grow in their distinctive culture, and develop perfect civilization.

(Swami Sivananda,
quoted in Max, 1970)

As I begin this afterword, I am perched on the top of a metaphorical hill, looking down. On the ground below, I see soil fertilized with neuroscience-based research, both on the effect of trauma on the nervous system and on the beneficial effects of various yoga practices. I see a tree with yogic roots taking hold in this rich medium. As I survey the trunk and branches, I see the yogic interventions described in this book, from hatha yoga postures to breathing practices, relaxation techniques, sense-withdrawal, and, finally, absorption in the quiet inner world of meditation. All of these resources create a balanced, yet dynamic, flow of energy, fortifying its practitioners for the challenges of remaining balanced, and of healing dysregulated somatic patterns, in a complex world.

Guarding the tree is a therapeutic fence which protects dysregulated clients, the seedlings, while they heal. Keeping the fence strong, but flexible, is a delicate practice for the therapist. It requires that the therapist practice self-care, to maintain a regulated ANS; be familiar enough with the interventions and their effects to know which one to choose; create an emotionally and physically safe environment for the client, so that learning and growth are possible; be tuned into the seedling's moment-to-moment experience in order to gauge the right intervention, at the right moment; and, finally, keep in mind the client's overall goals, directing each intervention toward their accomplishment.

From my high perch, in the far distance, I can see a variety of terrain, including large, bustling cities; pleasant towns; farms; local schools; colleges and universities; government offices, prisons, and military bases: the big picture. How these foundations of society function, including how ethical they are, what they value, and how responsive and resilient they are, plays a major role in the genesis of trauma, since humans internalize the behavior, attitudes, and beliefs to which they are exposed as they grow.

Currently, I see little awareness of the importance of physical and emotional safety, which supports nervous system regulation, in this landscape, and few resources built into its fabric to promote it. Using the NITYA Healing Model diagram to analyze contemporary American society, it seems that most people are in the overarousal zone, maintaining some degree of chronic fight and flight just to get through the day. This overactivation eventually must crash, taking its toll on the individual's health, and on the health of the culture at large, which are measures of quality of life.

I look forward to a time when the importance of maintaining ANS balance is recognized by the dominant culture, and its institutions and the way they treat people are reevaluated and restructured in that light. In the meantime, psychotherapists, yoga therapists, yoga instructors, and all teachers of meditative movement, are the harbingers of change, with much important work to do.

The quotation which opens this chapter emphasizes peace as the world's most important resource. A peaceful, safe, non-toxic environment is what trauma survivors need to heal; what healthy people need in order to maintain their health; and what the world needs in order to prosper. I maintain that yoga offers it, as a vision, and as a practical system. Its popularity and its current applications to the maintenance of mental health give me hope for the future.

The NITYA Healing Model

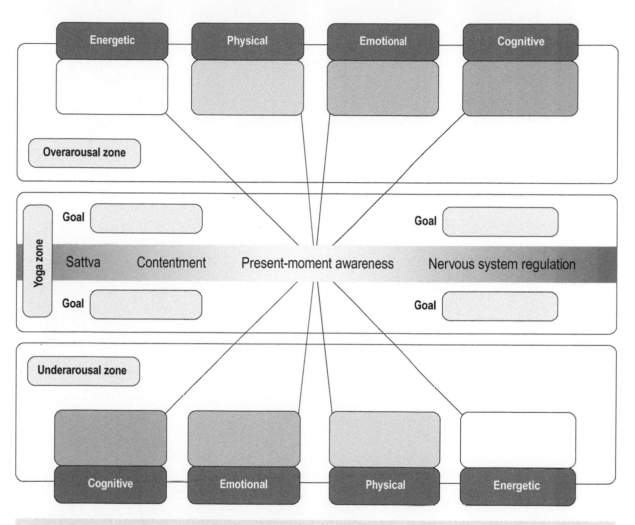

FIGURE A1.1 Blank NITYA healing chart for treatment planning.

Assessment tool

ASSESSMENT TOOL

1 Is the client open to a somatic intervention?

2 What is your treatment goal for bringing yoga into the session?

3 What is your analysis of the autonomic nervous system balance in the client (SNS/PNS overactivation; underactivation; both; no imbalance)?

4 Does the client have any medical condition which would limit, or benefit from, the practice?

5 Which yoga practice(s) would be most beneficial for that client (stretching, postures held in stillness, breath awareness, breathing practice, relaxation, meditation, or a combination)?

6 Which stage of the defense cascade is the client experiencing at this time?

7 What is the dominant energy state (guna) of the client: lethargic, hyper-energized, or stable and balanced?

8 Which symptoms of imbalance are you seeking to reduce?

9 Which interventions do you think would be most beneficial?

(Be as specific as possible.)

Moral/ethical_____

Physical postures_____

Breathing practices_____

Deep relaxation_____

Meditation_____

FIGURE A2.1 Assessment tool.

NITYA chair yoga script

The chair yoga warm-up and postures script

The focus in chair yoga is to enhance your ability to feel your body sensations and to tune more fully into your breath. All instructions are only guidelines. You are welcome to participate in a way that works for you. Please discontinue the practice if you feel pain.

Please take a comfortable seated position with your feet touching the floor (you can use a pillow or block under your feet if necessary), your spine as straight as possible, and your hands resting on your knees or thighs. You are welcome to pause and take a breath. Notice the points of contact between the back of your body and the chair and the soles of your feet and the floor. You are invited to tune in to the natural flow of your breath, watching it as it flows in and out, and not trying to change it, for three breaths.

You are now welcome to do some arm breathing, raising your arms as you inhale and lowering them as you exhale. Please continue that for three breaths, on your own. As you exhale you may feel yourself sinking a little bit deeper into the chair.

Joint warm-up (these are not yoga postures, but, rather, prepare the body for the postures)

You are invited to rotate the major joints of the body, warming them up for the postures. You can start by rotating your fingers, then the wrists, in both directions. (Pause.) You can then move your awareness up the arm and slowly rotate the elbows, first in one direction and then the other, and then the shoulders. You can now let that movement go. How is your breathing? (Pause.) Making slow movements, as you inhale, you can raise the shoulders toward the ears. Then you can press them down toward the feet, exhaling. Pause for an inhale. On the next exhale, you can squeeze the shoulders together toward the center of the chest. When you are ready, on an inhale, arch the spine and bring the shoulders toward the center of the back. Then you can release the shoulders, bring your spine back to neutral, and pause to take a breath.

Now you are invited to move your awareness to the toes and feet. You may want to remove your shoes. You can stretch the toes, then rotate the ankles in both directions. Pause to take a breath. You can move your awareness up your legs to the knees. Inhale as you raise the right leg, and exhale as you lower it. Do the same thing with the left leg. Now, if you are able, on your next inhale, raise both legs at the same time, continuing to breathe. Hold them as long as you comfortably can (up to 10 seconds), and then release them. Pause to take three breaths.

You are now invited to explore the range of motion in the spine, first, on the inhale, arching it, bringing the shoulder blades closer together, toward the center of the back. Slowly continue this backward curving motion with the neck and head, raising them an inch or two. Then you are welcome to do the opposite on the exhale, flexing the spine into a c-shape and curving the neck and head forward. Feel free to continue exploring these movements in coordination with the breath. (Pause.)

Now, bring your awareness to your waist. On your next inhale, begin rotating the torso, from the waist, in a clockwise direction, over the seated hips. What sensations do you notice? (Pause.) Now rotate the torso in the other direction. (Pause.) You can come back to center and take three breaths.

Moving your awareness up the body, you can focus on relaxing the neck. You are welcome to slowly nod your head *yes*. You can inhale as you raise it, and exhale as you lower it. Then you can shake your head *no*, moving the head slowly from side to side, moving through center. Let your breath set the pace. (Pause.) Come back to stillness. Now, as you exhale, let your right ear tilt toward the right shoulder. Take three breaths in that position, if that is comfortable. Now straighten your head and let the left ear tilt toward the left shoulder. You can exhale as the head tilts and inhale as it straightens. You are welcome to repeat this movement a few times. (Pause.)

Feel free to make any other movements to relax your body a little bit more. Notice any changes in your body sensations and breath as a result of the warm-up.

The eye movements

(NOTE: This section of the script incorporates instructions from Stanley Rosenberg, *Accessing the Healing Power of the Vagus Nerve*, North Atlantic Books, 2017. With permission of North Atlantic Books.) Sit in a comfortable position, with your hands on your lap or knees, head facing straight ahead. Begin the first round of the eye movements by inhaling. Keeping your head still during this round, on the exhale, look to the far-right corner of your vision. (Pause for three breaths.) Repeat

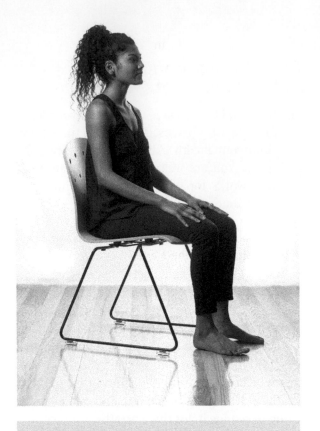

FIGURE A3.1 Simple seated pose.

this movement, bringing your gaze to the far left. (Again, pause.) Now look upward. (Pause.) Next, look down toward the floor, and pause. Now bring your gaze back to center. You can rub your palms together briskly, building up heat, and gently cup your hands over your eyes, with your fingertips in your hairline, until the heat dissipates.

In the second round, take a breath, then again look to the far-right corner of your vision. This time, leaving your gaze there, turn your head to the left and hold that position for up to 30 seconds, or until you swallow, yawn, or sigh. Release the head and eyes, and repeat the exercise in the other direction, bringing your gaze to the far left, and turning your head to the right. Again, hold for up to 30 seconds, or until you swallow, yawn, or sigh. Release the head and eyes, notice the points of contact between the back of your body and the chair, and the soles of your feet and the floor, and take a deep breath.

The chair poses

The first chair pose is a backward bending pose, the **cobra pose**. With the hands on the top of the thighs, you are invited to begin to slowly arch the spine and neck, opening the chest and compressing the shoulder blades toward the center of the back, raising the head an inch or two and looking up. (Pause.) If you are comfortable in the pose, you can hold it, and take three breaths. (Pause.) If your mind is wandering, please bring your awareness to the point between your shoulder blades. You can do this anytime the mind wanders. Notice the flow of the breath, and your body sensations. (Pause.)

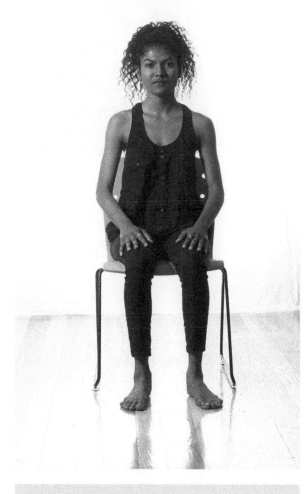

FIGURE A3.2 Seated cobra pose.

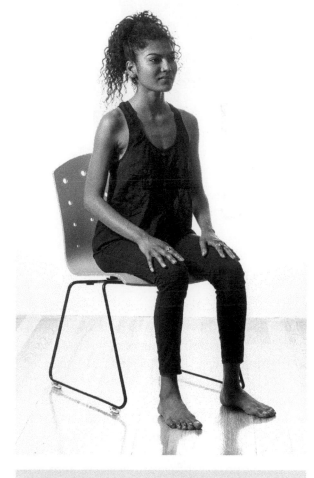

FIGURE A3.3 Forward bend, upright.

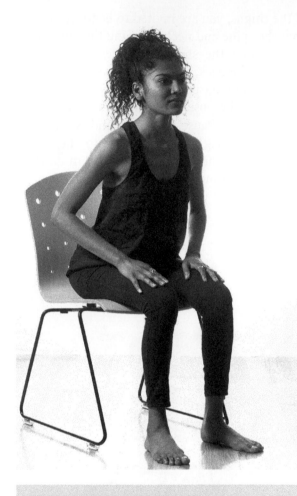

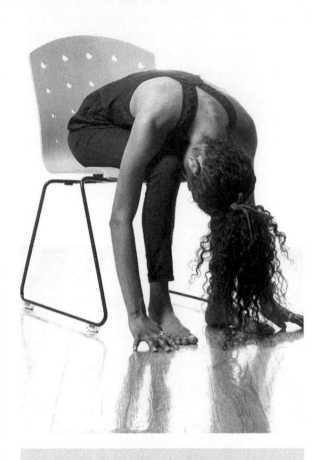

FIGURE A3.4 Forward bend, half-bent.

FIGURE A3.5 Forward bend, released.

You can come out of the pose by straightening the spine and bringing your head and neck back in alignment with it. After you have released the pose, you are invited to look around the room, letting your eyes go where they want to go. Bring the gaze back to center and watch the breath as it flows in and out.

The next pose is a **forward bending pose**, the full forward bend. Keeping the head as much in line with the spine as is possible, with the hands

on top the thighs, slowly bend forward from the waist, bringing the torso half-way down toward the legs. If you have a heart condition, uncontrolled high blood pressure or neck or head injuries, please hold the pose there.

If you don't, you are invited to slowly lower your torso closer to your legs, and, if you would like, let your head hang. Or you can hold it in line with the spine. Hold the pose as long as it is comfortable, focusing on the natural flow of

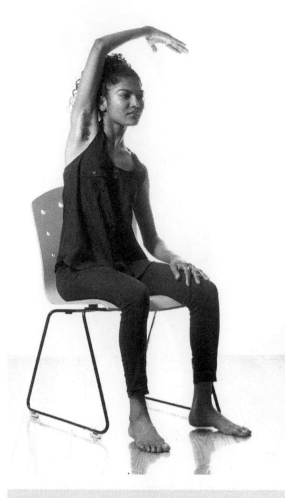

FIGURE A3.6 Half moon pose, right.

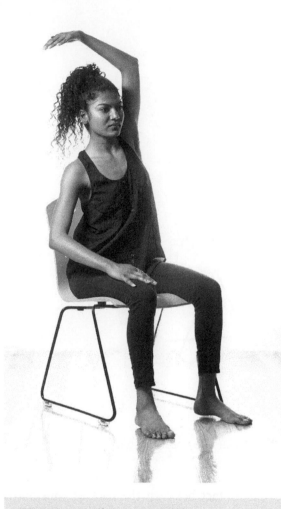

FIGURE A3.7 Half moon pose, left.

the breath. (Pause for 30 seconds, or until everyone is sitting up.) Slowly bring the head and neck back in line with the spine, and return to a seated position, with the hands on the top of the thighs. Please take three breaths.

We will now do the **seated half moon pose**. Sitting up straight, with the left hand on top of the left thigh, you are invited to slowly raise the right arm. With both buttocks on the chair, leading from the waist, lean the torso to the left. You

can let the right arm arc over your head. Please hold the pose and take three breaths. (Pause.) If your mind wanders, you can focus on a point under the raised arm. After your third exhale, straighten the torso and lower the arm by your side. Repeat the same pose to the right by raising the left arm, bending the torso toward the right, and making an arc over head with the left arm, continuing to breathe. (Pause.) When you are ready, straighten the torso and lower the left arm. You are welcome to take three breaths and

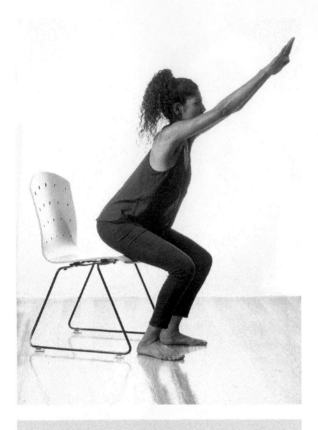

FIGURE A3.8 Chair pose, seated.

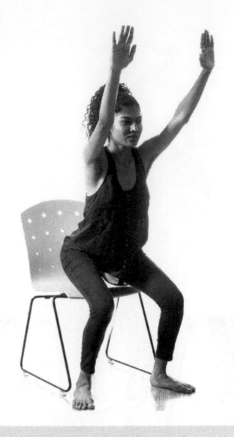

FIGURE A3.9 Chair pose, rising.

feel the contact between the back of your body and the chair, and the soles of your feet and the floor. (Pause.)

The next pose is the **chair pose**, which can build strength in the legs and core abdominal muscles. If you are dealing with a debilitating medical condition, or chronic SNS overactivation, you might want to opt out of this pose. If you are not, please put some weight on your feet and shift your center of gravity forward, as if you were going to stand. As you lift yourself a few inches off the chair, slowly raise the arms, so that the arms are straight and parallel, and the palms are facing each other. Your head, neck, and back can

be aligned at a 135-degree angle from the floor. Continue breathing while you hold the pose. This pose can be strenuous, so feel free to sit down when you begin to tire. (Have the client hold the pose for a maximum of 10 seconds.) Now sit and take three breaths. Notice the effect of this pose on your body and mind.

For the **half spinal twist**, sitting with your spine straight, you are invited to raise your arms overhead and twist to the right, starting at the waist and twisting the torso, shoulders, neck, and head. Gaze over the right shoulder. (Pause.) With the left hand, grasp the outside of the right thigh. Place your right hand on the

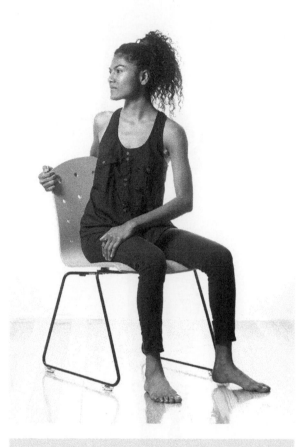

FIGURE A3.10 Half spinal twist, right.

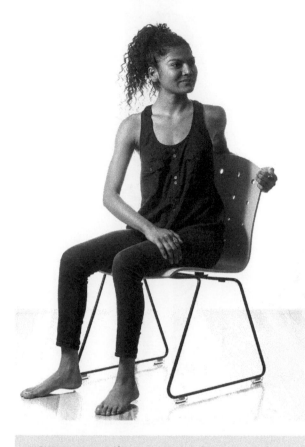

FIGURE A3.11 Half spinal twist, left.

seat or arm of the chair. Hold the pose and take three breaths, bringing your awareness to your entire spine. (Pause.) At the bottom of the third exhalation, feel free to twist to the right just a little bit more. On the inhale, please release the pose, untwisting the torso, arms, and legs, and returning to center.

You can repeat the posture on the left side. To begin, please raise the arms overhead and, starting at the waist, twist the torso to the left. Turning your head to the left, you can gaze over the left shoulder. Grasp the outside of the left

thigh with the right hand. Place your left hand on the seat or arm of the chair. You are welcome to hold the pose and take three breaths, focusing on your body sensations. (Pause.) At the bottom of the third exhalation, twist around a little farther to the left. On the next inhale, please release the pose, untwist the torso, arms, and legs, and return to center. Take a moment to experience your body sensations and breath. (Pause.)

The final posture is the **standing mountain pose**. Please stand with your weight evenly distributed over both feet. Feel the entire sole of each

121

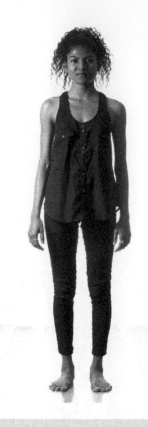

FIGURE A3.12 Mountain pose, standing.

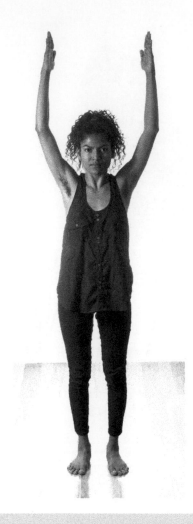

FIGURE A3.13 Mountain pose, arms raised here.

foot in contact with the floor. As much as possible, align your hips and shoulders over them, and have the neck in a straight line with the spine. Now you are invited to bring your arms overhead and parallel, with the palms facing each other. Take three breaths. (Pause.) Feel as if no one could ever move you from this spot unless you wanted to be moved.

After your next exhale, release the arms, and take a comfortable seated position, with your feet touching the floor, your spine straight and your hands resting on your thighs. Feel the points of contact between the back of your body and the chair, and the soles of your feet and the floor.

Watch the breaths for three breaths, and tune into your body sensations.

Notice if you feel different than you did before the practice. If so, note to yourself what the difference is. This is the end of our practice; thank you so much.

NITYA three-part deep breath script

Adapted from the Integral Yoga® Hatha Teacher Training manual ©2017 Satchidananda Ashram–Yogaville Inc. Used with permission.

Appendix 4

The yogic three-part deep breath is the basic breathing practice upon which the other breathing practices are built. It is composed of a slow, deep inhalation focusing on three segments of expansion, and a spontaneous exhale. This practice is calming and beneficial to the mind and body.

If you should feel uncomfortable in any way during this practice, such as experiencing light-headedness, dizziness, or the upwelling of emotions, please release the practice, and let the breath assume its natural flow. These symptoms are not serious, and usually pass quickly.

Take a moment to notice the natural flow of your breath. Watch the breath, accepting it exactly as it is, for three breaths. (Pause.) Now begin the practice with an exhale. At the bottom of the exhale, begin inhaling into the abdomen, feeling it expand like a big balloon. At the bottom of the exhale, begin inhaling into the abdomen, feeling it expand like a balloon. You can place your hands on the abdomen in order to feel the expansion. This is the first part of the three-part deep breath. The exhale should be done in the reverse order, exhaling from the chest, ribcage, and then the abdomen. Practice on your own for three breaths. (Pause.)

On your next inhalation, breathe into the abdomen, and then into the ribcage, feeling the ribs expand out to the side. You can imagine that the balloon is filled with helium, and it is rising up to the ribcage. Again, you are welcome to place

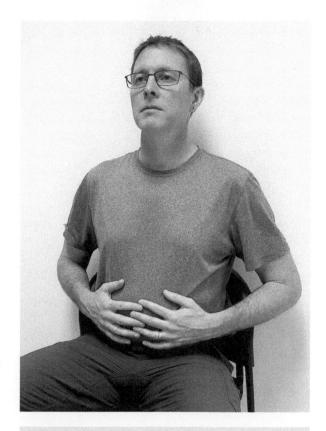

Figure A4.1 Three-part deep breath, hands on abdomen.

your hands on your ribs to feel the expansion, and exhale in the opposite order of the inhalation. This is the second part of the deep breath; practice on your own for three breaths. (Pause.)

Now inhale into the abdomen and the ribcage, and bring the air into the chest, expanding the upper chest. Can you feel the collar bones rise

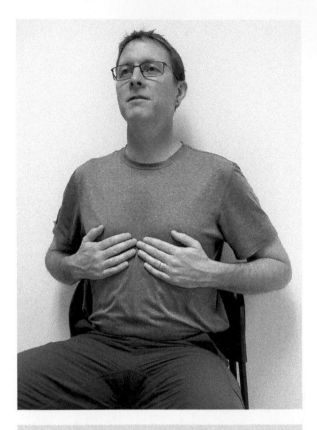

Figure A4.2 Three-part deep breath, hands on ribcage.

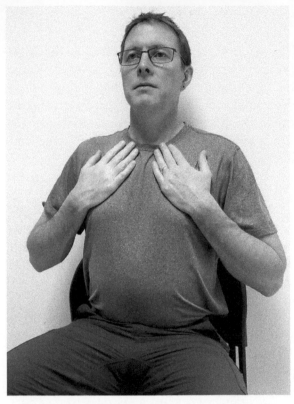

Figure A4.3 Three-part breath, hands on upper chest.

slightly? Again, you can use the image of a helium balloon expanding to fill your chest. You can place your hands on the abdomen if you would like to feel the expansion. This is the last part of the three-part deep breath. Exhale in the opposite order of the inhale: chest, ribcage, and then the abdomen. Practice on your own for three breaths. (Pause.)

Finally, you can combine the three parts into one smooth breath. Practice that for three breaths.

(Pause.) After the third exhale, allow the breath to return to normal, and observe any changes which may have taken place in your body and/or mind.

Alternate nostril breathing

Alternate nostril breathing is the three-part deep breath done by inhaling and exhaling through one nostril at a time. To begin, please make a gentle fist with the right hand, then release the thumb and last

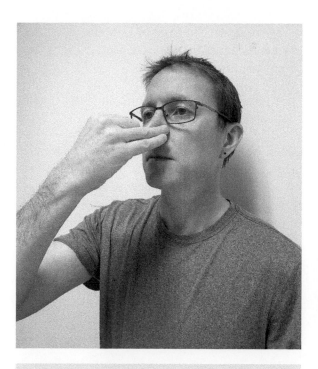

Figure A4.4 Alternate nostril breathing, left nostril closed.

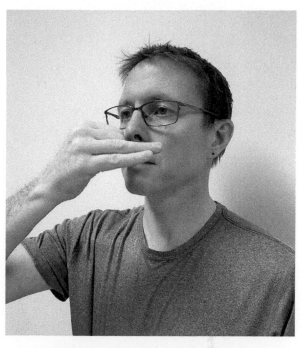

Figure A4.5 Alternate nostril breathing, right nostril closed.

two fingers. At the top of your next inhale, close off the right nostril with the thumb, and exhale slowly through the left. Breathe slowly and deeply, without strain. Inhale slowly through the left, close it off with the last two fingers, release the thumb, and exhale through the right. Inhale through the right, close it off, and exhale through the left. Continue to breathe in this pattern, exhaling and inhaling through the same nostril, then switching. (Pause.)

After your next exhalation through the right nostril, release the practice, bring your hand to your lap, and let the breath return to normal.

Brahmari

To begin the practice of brahmari, please inhale through the nostrils, filling the lungs completely. Then exhale while making a humming sound, with the lips shut and the tongue relaxed and in contact with the roof of the mouth. This practice vibrates in the head. Please note where you most feel the vibration.

SCRIPT

Padadhirasana script (breath balancing pose)

Please sit in a comfortable position.

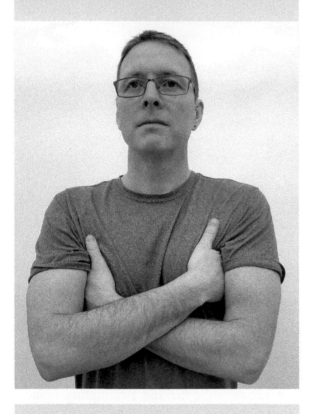

Figure A4.6 Padadhirasana.

Cross your arms in front of your chest, placing your hands under the opposite armpits, with the thumbs pointing upward.

The point between the thumb and first finger should be firmly pressed.

Become aware of your breath (pause); you are welcome to close your eyes if that feels right. For as long as is comfortable, take slow, deep, rhythmical breaths, until you sense that the flow of breath in both nostrils is equalized. Notice how that feels.

SCRIPT

Part one: progressive deep relaxation *(for all clients)*

I am going to lead you through yoga nidra, the yogic sleep, into a state of deep relaxation. You can sit or lie down, and have your eyes open or closed, whatever is more comfortable for you. Feel free to interrupt me at any time if you have a question or problem by raising your hand, and please discontinue the practice at any time if you feel uncomfortable.

(Speaking slowly.) You are invited to notice the points of contact between the back of your body and surface you are relaxing on. (Pause.) Tune into the natural flow of your breath. (Pause.) Now, bring your awareness to your right foot and leg. Stretch out the toes, then tense the muscles of the foot and leg. *(Increase the intensity of your voice.)* Raise it a few inches off the floor, hold, squeeze, then let it gently fall back to the floor. Roll the leg from side to side and let it go. (Pause.) Focus on the breath for two breaths.

Now stretch out the toes of your left foot. *(Increase the intensity of your voice.)* Tense the muscles of the foot and leg. Raise it a few inches off the floor … holding, tightening … then release it. Roll it from side to side and let it go. (Pause.) Again, focus on the breath.

Focusing on your right hand, stretch out the fingers, then make a fist. *(Increase the intensity of your voice.)* Tense the muscles of the right hand and arm and raise it a few inches. Hold … tense … relax, and release. Roll it from side to side, and let it go. (Pause.) Notice the breath.

Focusing on your left hand, stretch out the fingers, then make a fist. *(Increase the intensity of your voice.)* Continue by tensing it, raising, and holding. Release the arm, rolling it from side to side, and let it go. (Pause.) Focus on the breath for two breaths.

Focusing on the buttock muscles, the ones you sit on, squeeze them together. *(Increase the intensity of your voice.)* Hold, tighten, and let them go. Roll the hips gently from side to side. (Pause.)

Focus on the breath. After your next exhalation, inhale deeply through the nose, into the abdomen, blowing it up like a balloon. *(Increase the intensity of your voice.)* Take in a little more air, a little more, and, through an open mouth, release it! Now, inhale into the chest, filling the chest with air. *(Increase the intensity of your voice.)* Take in a little more air, a little more, then, through an open mouth, release it! Let the breath return to normal and watch it for three breaths. (Pause.)

Bring your awareness to your shoulders. First, as you exhale, squeeze the shoulders together toward the center of the chest. Hold, squeeze, and release. Then, as you inhale, compress the shoulder blades toward the center of the back, feeling the chest expand and the back arching. Release the shoulders as you exhale. (Pause.) Now, as you inhale, raise the shoulders, as if to touch the ears. Squeeze, and release. Then, exhaling, press them down toward the feet, and release them.

Gently roll the head from side to side, as you watch the breath. (Pause.)

Open your mouth and roll the jaw around. (Pause.) Now close your mouth and, as you inhale, suck in the cheeks, and pucker the lips. Exhale, and release. (Pause.) As you inhale, tense the muscles of the nostrils, and release with an exhalation. Inhale, knitting the eyebrows together in the center of your forehead; exhale and release. Inhale again, raising the eyebrows toward the top of the head. Exhale and release. (Pause.) Take a breath.

Now, as you inhale, make your face as long as you can by opening your mouth, sticking out your tongue, pointing it toward your feet, and looking up toward the top of your head. Release. Now do just the opposite: inhale as you bring all of the facial features together into a ball in the center of the face. Squeeze … and release. Do that one more time, and release. Again, gently roll the head from side to side, and bring it back to center. Please take a breath. (Pause.)

Part two: body scan *(for clients who are comfortable with, and are able to do, a mental scan of their body parts while continuing to breathe)*

Now that you have relaxed the major muscles of the body, you can use the power of suggestion, the power of the mind, to relax the body a little bit more. Without moving, except for the flow of the breath, bring your awareness to your toes (pause), soles of the feet (pause), and tops of the feet (pause), sending them a mental suggestion

to release a little bit more. (Brief pause after each body part named.) Release the lower legs, knees, upper legs, buttocks muscles, and finally the entire pelvis. Please take a breath. (Pause.)

Bring your awareness to your hands. (Brief pause after each body part named.) Release muscular tension in the fingers, palms, back of the hands, lower arms, elbows, upper arms, and shoulders. (Pause.) Take a breath. Now, bring your awareness to the abdominal area. Release muscular tension in the abdominal organs, ribcage, lungs, and chest. Please take a breath. (Pause.)

(Brief pause after each body part named.) Bring your awareness to your back. Release tension in the lower back, middle back, and upper back, feeling every point of contact between your back and surface you are resting on. (Pause.)

(Brief pause after each body part named.) Relax the throat, jaw, cheeks, lips, teeth, and even the tongue. Relax the nose, eyes, eyebrows, forehead, and scalp. Please take a breath. (Pause.)

Part three: visualizing peaceful energy *(for clients with good body awareness who can lie still for a few minutes and are comfortable with a visualization exercise)*

(Speak slowly and softly.) Feel that your scalp is being bathed in a peaceful energy which is slowly spreading down the torso, arms, and legs, revitalizing and rejuvenating every cell. (One minute of complete silence.)

Part four: silent witnessing *(for clients experienced in yoga and in trauma therapy who are not consciously engaging in injurious behavior toward themselves or others)*

Now bring your awareness to your breath. Watch the breath as it flows in and out. Don't try to control it; just watch. Be a silent witness to the flow of the breath. (Pause 30 seconds.) Continue to watch the breath. (30 seconds of complete silence.)

Now shift your awareness to your thoughts. Don't be attached to them, just watch them, as if you were watching a movie. (Pause 30 seconds.) Continue the watch the thoughts. (30 seconds of complete silence.)

Now see if you can find a place that is deeper than the thoughts, a place where there are no thoughts. If you find this peaceful place, just enjoy it. If not, you can watch the thoughts, or watch the breath. (Five minutes of complete silence.)

Bring your awareness back to your breath, deepening it. (Pause.) Start to wake the body by moving the fingers and toes, arms, and legs. When you are ready, you can open your eyes, roll onto your right side, and slowly sit up. (Pause.) Now look around the room, letting your eyes go where they want to go, until they come back to centered gaze. This is the end of the yoga nidra practice.

Abbreviations

ACE study	Adverse Childhood Experiences study
ANB	alternate nostril breathing
ANS	autonomic nervous system
CNS	central nervous system
CO_2	carbon dioxide
DMN	default mode network
DSM	Diagnostic and Statistical Manual of Mental Disorders
DVC	dorsal (back) vagal complex
EEG	electroencephalogram
EMDR	eye movement desensitization and reprocessing
HRV	heart rate variability
ICD	International Classification of Disease
NITYA	Nervous System-Informed, Trauma-Sensitive Yoga (NITYA) Healing Model
NO	nitric oxide
PNS	parasympathetic nervous system
PTSD	post-traumatic stress disorder
SNS	sympathetic nervous system
VVC	ventral (front) vagal complex
WOT	window of tolerance

Bibliography

Abrams MP, Carleton RN, Taylor S, Asmundson GJG. Human tonic immobility: measurement and correlates. Depress Anxiety. 2009;26(6):550–6. doi: 10.1002/da.20462

Alves PN, Foulon C, Karolis V, Bzdok D, Volle E, Schotten MT de. An improved neuroanatomical model of the default-mode network reconciles previous neuroimaging and neuropathological findings. Communications Biology. 2019; vol. 2, article 370.

American Psychiatric Association. Diagnostic and Statistical Manual of Mental Disorders, Fifth Edition (DSM-5). Washington DC: American Psychiatric Publishing; 2013.

American Psychiatric Association. Diagnostic and Statistical Manual of Mental Disorders. New Delhi: CBS Publishers; 2017.

Anderson S. Guide to agni sara. Yoga International; 2013 [accessed 15 October 2020]. Available from: https://yogainternational.com/article/view/guide-to-agni-sara.

Ashok HS, Thimmappa MS. A Hindu worldview of adult learning in the workplace. Advances in Developing Human Resources, 2006;8(3):330–1. doi:10.1177/1523422306288425

Avalon A. Serpent power – the secrets of tantric and shaktic yoga. Mineola, NY: Dover Publications; 1974.

Beauchaine T. Vagal tone, development, and Gray's motivational theory: Toward an integrated model of autonomic nervous system functioning in psychopathology. Development and Psychopathology. 2001;13(2):183–214. doi:10.1017/s0954579401002012.

Berkovich-Ohana A, Wilf M, Kahana R, Arieli A, Malach R. Repetitive speech elicits widespread deactivation in the human cortex: the "mantra" effect? Brain Behaviour. 2015;5(7):e00346.

Bernardi L, Sleight P, Bandinelli G, Cencetti S, Fattorini L, Wdowczyc-Szulc J, Lagi A. Effect of rosary prayer and yoga mantras on autonomic cardiovascular rhythms: comparative study. BMJ. 2001;323(7327):1446–9.

Berntson GG, Norman GJ, Hawkley LC, Cacioppo JT. Cardiac autonomic balance versus cardiac regulatory capacity. Psychophysiology. 2008;45(4):643–52. doi:10.1111/j.1469-8986.2008.00652.

Bharati SV. Yogi in the lab: Future directions of scientific research in meditation. Rishikesh, India: AHMSIN Publishing; 2006.

Bharati SV. Chronic nostril dominance. Swami Veda Bharati; 2012 [accessed 22 January 2018]. Available from: https://www.scribd.com/document/264749600/Chronic-Nostril-Dominance

Bharati SV. My Experiments with Yoga Nidra. Rishikesh, India: Himalayan Yoga Publications Trust; 2014.

Bhavanani A, Ramanathan M. Nasal cycle and its therapeutic applications: a yogic perspective. Proceedings at National Conference on Chronobiology and Health; 2016 [accessed 2 Aug. 2019]. Available from: https://www.researchgate.net/publication/299215358_Nasal_cycle_and_its_therapeutic_applications_a_yogic_perspective

Bhavanani AB, Raj JB, Ramanathan M, Trakroo M. Effect of different pranayamas on respiratory sinus arrhythmia. Journal of Clinical and Diagnostic Research. 2016;10(3): CC04–6. doi:10.7860/jcdr/2016/16306.7408

Birch J, Hargreaves J. Yoganidra: an understanding of the history and context. The Luminescent; 2015 [accessed 19 October 2020]. Available from: http://theluminescent.blogspot.co.uk/2015_01_01_archive.html.

Blake DD, Weathers FW, Nagy LM, Kaloupek DG, Gusman FD, Charney DS, Keane TM. The development of a clinician-administered PTSD scale. Journal of Traumatic Stress. 1995;8:75–90.

Blechert J, Michael T, Grossman P, Lajtman M, Wilhelm FH. Autonomic and respiratory characteristics of post-traumatic stress disorder and panic disorder. Psychosomatic Medicine. 2007;69(9):935–43. doi:10.1097/psy.0b013e31815a8f6b

Bloom S. Creating sanctuary: Toward the Evolution of Sane Societies. Routledge; 2nd ed., 2013.

Bolger EP, Judson MA. The therapeutic value of singing. New England Journal of Medicine. 1984;311(26):1704. doi: 10.1056/nejm198412273112621

Brandani JZ, Mizuno J, Ciolac EG, Monteiro HL. The hypotensive effect of Yoga's breathing exercises:

A systematic review. Complementary Therapies in Clinical Practice. 2017;28:38–46 [accessed 1 Aug. 2019]. Available from: https://www.sciencedirect.com/science/article/pii/S174438811730172X doi:10.1016/j.ctcp.2017.05.002.

Bremner JD. Traumatic stress: effects on the brain. Dialogues in Clinical Neuroscience. 2006;8(4):445–61.

Brown RP, Gerbarg PL. The Healing Power of the Breath: Simple Techniques to Reduce Stress and Anxiety, Enhance Concentration, and Balance Your Emotions. Boulder, CO: Shambhala; 2012.

Calancie OG, Khalid-Khan S, Booij L, Munoz DP. Eye movement desensitization and reprocessing as a treatment for PTSD: current neurobiological theories and a new hypothesis. Annals of the New York Academy of Sciences. 2018;1426(1):127–45. https://doi.org/10.1111/nyas.13882

Cardeña E, Carlson EB. Acute stress disorder revisited. Annual Review of Clinical Psychology. 2011;7:245–67.

Cognitive therapy. Wikipedia; 2017 [accessed 27 January 2018]. Available from: https://en.wikipedia.org/w/index.php?title=Cognitive_therapy&oldid=812923840.

Conrad A, Roth WT. Muscle relaxation therapy for anxiety disorders: it works, but how? Journal of Anxiety Disorders. 2007;21(3):243–64. doi: 10.1016/j.janxdis.2006.08.001.

Coulter HD. Chapter 5. In: Anatomy of Hatha Yoga: A manual for students, teachers, and practitioners. Honesdale, PA: Body and Breath; 2012.

Cozolino L. It's a jungle in there: we're not as evolved as we think. Psychotherapy Networker. 2008;32(5): October.

Cozolino L. The neuroscience of psychotherapy: healing the social brain. 2nd ed. New York: W. W. Norton & Company; 2010.

Damasio AR. Descartes' error: emotion, reason, and the human brain. Kindle edition. London: Penguin Books; 2005.

Davidson RJ, Kabat-Zinn J, Schumacher J, Rosenkranz M, Muller D, Santorelli SF, Urbanowski F, Harrington A, Bonus K, Sheridan JF. Alterations in brain and immune function produced by mindfulness meditation. Psychosomatic Medicine. 2003;65(4), pp.564–570.

Davies AM, Eccles R. Reciprocal changes in nasal resistance to airflow caused by pressure applied to the axilla. Acta Oto-Laryngologica. 1985;99(1–2):154–9.

Desai K. Yoga Nidra: The art of transformational sleep. Twin Lakes, WI: Lotus Press; 2017. 10

Devi NJ. The secret power of yoga: a woman's guide to the heart and spirit of the yoga sutras. New York: Three Rivers Press; 2007.

Dhanvijay A, Chandan L. Effect of Nadi Shuddhi Pranayama on perceived stress and cardiovascular autonomic functions in 1st year undergraduate medical students. National Journal of Physiology, Pharmacy and Pharmacology. 2018;8(6):898–902. doi:10.5455/njppp.2018.8.0205515022018.

Dillon WC, Hampl V, Shultz PJ, Rubins JB, Archer SL. Origins of breath nitric oxide in humans. Chest. October 1996;110(4):930–8.

Doidge N. The brain that changes itself: stories of personal triumph from the frontiers of brain science. New York: Viking; 2007.

Dykema R. Don't talk to me now, I'm scanning for danger: How your nervous system sabatoges your ability to relate: An interview with Stephen Porges about his polyvagal theory. Nexus. 2006:30–35.

Easwaran E. Introduction. In: The Bhagavad Gita. 2nd ed. Tomales, CA: Nilgiri Press; 2007; 43–7.

Elliott S. The new science of breath: Coherent breathing for autonomic nervous system balance, health, and wellbeing. Allen, TX: Coherence Press; 2005.

Emerson D, Sharma R, Chaudry S, Turner J. Yoga therapy in practice: trauma-sensitive yoga: principles, practice, and research. International Journal of Yoga Therapy. 2009;19:123–8.

Emerson D, Hopper E, van der Kolk B, Levine PA, Cope S. Overcoming trauma through yoga: reclaiming your body. 1 edition ed. Berkeley, CA: North Atlantic Books; 2011.

Felitti VJ, Anda RF, Nordenberg D, Williamson DF, Spitz AM, Edwards V, Koss MP, Marks JS. Relationship of childhood abuse and household dysfunction to many of the leading causes of death in adults. The Adverse

Childhood Experiences (ACE) Study. American Journal of Preventative Medicine. 1998;14(245–58).

Fenn K, Byrne M. The key principles of cognitive behavioural therapy. InnovAiT: Education and Inspiration for General Practice. 2013;6(9):579–85. [accessed 20 October 2020]. doi:10.1177/1755738012471029. Available from: https://journals.sagepub.com/doi/full/10.1177/1755738012471029.

Flatten G, Perlitz V, Pestinger M, Arin T, Kohl B, Kastrau F, Schnitker R, Vohn R, Weber J, Ohnhaus M, Petzold ER, Erli HJ. Neural processing of traumatic events in subjects suffering PTSD – a case study of two surgical patients with severe accident trauma. GMS Psycho-Social Medicine. 2004;1:Doc06 [accessed 28 January 2018]. Available from: https://www.ncbi.nlm.nih.gov/pmc/articles/PMC2736480

Frawley D. Ayurveda and the mind: the healing of consciousness. Twin Lakes, WI: Lotus Press; 1997.

Frawley D, Kozak SS. Yoga for your type: an ayurvedic approach to your asana practice. Twin Lakes, WI: Lotus Press; 2001.

Frawley D, Kozak SS, Farmer A. Chapter 8: Ayurvedic Effects of Asana Practice. In: Yoga for your type: An ayurvedic approach to your asana practice. Twin Lakes, WI: Lotus Press; 2001: 33.

Freud S. [1905]. Fragment of an analysis of a case of hysteria ("Dora"). In: The Freud Reader, P. Gay (Ed.). London: Vintage; 1995.

Furness JB, Callaghan BP, Rivera LR, Cho HJ. The enteric nervous system and gastrointestinal innervation: integrated local and central control. Advances in Experimental Medicine & Biology. 2014;817:39–71. doi: 10.1007/978-1-4939-0897-4_3.

Gangadhar B, Kalyani B, Venkatasubramanian G, Arasappa R, Rao N, Kalmady S, Behere RV, Rao H, Vasudev, M, Gangadhar BN. Neurohemodynamic correlates of 'OM' chanting: A pilot functional magnetic resonance imaging study. International Journal of Yoga. 2011;4(1):3. doi:10.4103/0973-6131.78171.

Gard T, Noggle JJ, Park CL, Vago DR, Wilson A. Potential self-regulatory mechanisms of yoga for psychological health. Frontiers in Human Neuroscience. 2014;8:770 [accessed 20 January 2018]. Available from: https://www.frontiersin.org/articles/10.3389/fnhum.2014.00770/full.

Gillig MG, Sanders RD. Cranial Nerves IX, X, XI, and XII. Psychiatry (Edgmont). 2010;7(5):37–41.

Gottschal T, Waal Malefijt MD. Nose breathing (swara-yoga). In: Migraines and headaches: Causes and solutions. Zuid-Scharwoude: Gottswaal VOF; 2019.

Green E, Green A. Beyond biofeedback. 1st ed. New York: Delacorte Press/S. Lawrence; 1977.

Grof C, Grof S. The stormy search for the self: A guide to personal growth through transformational crisis. New York: Putnams; 1992.

Halpern, M. Ayurvedic Yoga Therapy Course, unpublished course manual.

Hanson R. Buddha's brain: the practical neuroscience of happiness, love & wisdom. Unabridged ed. Grand Haven, MI: Brilliance Audio; 2014.

Harne BP, Hiwale AS. EEG Spectral analysis on om mantra meditation: a pilot study. Applied Psychophysiology and Biofeedback. 2018;43(2):123–9. doi:10.1007/s10484-018-9391-7.

Hebb D. The organization of behavior. Abingdon, UK: Psychology Press; 2002.

Herrero JL, Khuvis S, Yeagle E, Cerf M, Mehta AD. Breathing above the brain stem: volitional control and attentional modulation in humans. Journal of Neurophysiology. 2018;119(1):145–59. doi: 10.1152/jn.00551.2017.

Herrmann N. What is the function of the various brainwaves? Scientific American. 1997 [accessed 20 October 2020] Available at: https://www.scientificamerican.com/article/what-is-the-function-of-t-1997-12-22/.

Holden C. Paul MacLean and the triune brain. Science. 1979;204(4397):1066–8.

Hoskinson S, Thunell A. (2019) The end of trauma workbook: A 10-week course of Trauma Safe™ tools for health and resilience. Encinitas: Organic Intelligence; 2019.

Hoskinson S. Somatic Experiencing Level 1, training notes.

"How do you feel? Lecture by Bud Craig." Vimeo, December 14, 2009 [accessed 20 October 2020]. Uploaded by Medicinska fakulteten vid LiU. Available from: https://vimeo.com/8170544.

Howes R. The polyvagal circuit in the consulting room: A interview with Stephen Porges. Psychotherapy Networker. 2013 [accessed 20 October 2020]. Available from: https://www.psychotherapynetworker.org/blog/details/105/the-polyvagal-circuit-in-the-consulting-room.

Huang EJ, Reichardt LF. Neurotrophins: roles in neuronal development and function. Annual Review of Neuroscience. 2001;24:677–736.

Iyengar BKS. Light on yoga. New York: Schocken Books; 1978.

Iyengar BKS, Rivers-Moore D. Yoga vrksa: the tree of yoga. Oxford: Fine Line; 1988.

Jerath R, Edry JW, Barnes VA, Jerath V. Physiology of long pranayamic breathing: neural respiratory elements may provide a mechanism that explains how slow deep breathing shifts the autonomic nervous system. Medical Hypotheses. 2006;67(3):566–71.

Jerath R, Crawford MW, Barnes VA, Harden, K. Self-regulation of breathing as a primary treatment for anxiety. Applied Psychophysiology and Biofeedback, 2015;40(2):107–15. doi:10.1007/s10484-015-9279-8.

Johnson CV, Friedman HL. Enlightened or delusional? Journal of Humanistic Psychology. 2008;48(4):505–27. doi:10.1177/0022167808314174

Johnson SL. Resources for improved coping. In: Therapist's Guide to Posttraumatic Stress Disorder Intervention. London: Elsevier; 2009:251–346.

Kaoverii, Twists, extensions and coasting with the vagal brake, Subtle Yoga, 16 October 2018. https://subtleyoga.com/why-are-flexion-and-twists-useful-for-anxiety-and-extensions-and-side-bends-good-for-depression/

Kesarcodi-Watson I. Samādhi in Patañjali's Yoga Sūtras (pp. 78). Philosophy East and West, 1982;32(1):77–90. doi:10.2307/1398753.

Keuning J. On the nasal cycle. Journal of International Rhinology, 1968;6:99–136.

Khan K. How somatic therapy can help patients suffering from psychological trauma. Psych Central; 2014. [accessed 28 January 2018]. Available from: https://psychcentral.com/blog/how-somatic-therapy-can-help-patients-suffering-from-psychological-trauma/

Khattab K, Khattab AA, Ortak J, Richardt G, Bonnemeier H. Iyengar yoga increases cardiac parasympathetic nervous modulation among healthy yoga practitioners. Evidence-based Complementary and Alternative Medicine. 2007;4(4):511–7.

Khemka SS, Ramarao NH, Hankey A. Effect of integral yoga on psychological and health variables and their correlations. International Journal of Yoga. 2011;4(2):93–9. doi:10.4103/0973-6131.85492.

Kjaer TW, Bertelsen C, Piccini P, Brooks D, Alving J, Lou HC. Increased dopamine tone during meditation-induced change of consciousness. Brain Research: Cognitive Brain Research. 2002;13(2):255–9.

Kozlowska K, Walker P, McLean L, Carrive P. Fear and the defense cascade: clinical implications and management. Harvard Review of Psychiatry. 2015;23(4), 263–287. doi:10.1097/HRP.0000000000000065.

Kraftsow G. Yoga for transformation: ancient teachings and holistic practices for healing body, mind, and heart. New York: Penguin Compass; 2002.

Krama. Yogapedia; 2018 [accessed 22 January 2018]. Available from: https://www.yogapedia.com/definition/5691/krama

Kuppusamy M, Kamaldeen D, Pitani R, Amaldas J, Shanmugam P. Effects of bhramari pranayama on health – A systematic review. Journal of Traditional Complementary Medicine. 2017;18;8(1):11–16. doi: 10.1016/j.jtcme.2017.02.003

Levine PA. Waking the tiger. Berkeley, CA: North Atlantic Books; 1997.

Levine PA. In an unspoken voice: how the body releases trauma and restores goodness. Berkeley, CA: North Atlantic Books; 2010.

Levine PA. Trauma and memory. Berkeley, CA: North Atlantic Books; 2015.

Lindahl JR, Fisher NE, Cooper DJ, Rosen RK, Britton WB. The varieties of contemplative experience: A mixed-methods study of meditation-related challenges in Western Buddhists. PLOS ONE. 2017;12(5):e0176239.

Loizzo, Joseph, interview with Stephen Porges, https://nalandainstitute.org/2018/04/17/loves-brain-a-conversation-with-stephen-porges/

Lukoff D, Lu F, Turner R. From spiritual emergency to spiritual problem: the transpersonal roots of the new DSM-IV category. Journal of Humanistic Psychology. 1998;38(2):21–50. doi:10.1177/00221678980382003

Lundberg JO. Nitric oxide and the paranasal sinuses. Anatomical Record (Hoboken). 2008;291(11):1479–84. doi: 10.1002/ar.20782.

McCraty R, Shaffer F. Heart rate variability: new perspectives on physiological mechanisms, assessment of self-regulatory capacity, and health risk. Global Advances in Health and Medicine. 2015;4(1):46–61. doi:10.7453/gahmj.2014.073

McFarlane AC, Yehuda R, Clark CR. Biologic models of traumatic memories and post-traumatic stress disorder. The role of neural networks. The Psychiatric Clinics of North America. 2002;25(2):253–270, v.

Manalai P, Hamilton RG, Langenberg P, Kosisky SE, Lapidus M, Sleemi A, Scrandis D, Cabassa JA, Rogers CA, Regenold WT, Dickerson F, Vittone BJ, Guzman A, Balis T, Tonelli LH, Postolache TT. Pollen-specific immunoglobulin E positivity is associated with worsening of depression scores in bipolar disorder patients during high pollen season. Bipolar Disorders. 2012;14(1):90–8. doi:10.1111/j.1399-5618.2012.00983.x.

Mangalteertham S. 1998. Yoga nidra – altered state of consciousness. In: Swami Satyananda. Yoga nidra. 6th ed. Chennai: Nesma Books; 2003.

Marlock G, Weiss H, Young C, Soth M. (eds.) The handbook of body psychotherapy and somatic psychology. Berkeley, CA: North Atlantic Books; 2015.

Max P. Peace. New York: William Morrow & Co.; 1970.

Mayo Clinic on Dissociative disorders. 2017 [accessed 27 October 2020]. Available from: https://www.mayoclinic.org/diseases-conditions/dissociative-disorders/symptoms-causes/syc-20355215

MedicineNet. Medical definition of peripheral nervous system. MedicineNet; 2018 [accessed 20 January 2018]. Available from: <https://www.medicinenet.com/script/main/art.asp?articlekey=8258>

Miller R. Chapter 2: The practice of yoga nidra. In: Yoga nidra: Awaken to unqualified presence through traditional mind-body practices. Louisville, CO: Sounds True; 2012.

Miller-Karas E. Building resilience to trauma: the trauma and community resiliency models. 1st ed. New York: Routledge; 2015.

Mishra RS (also known as Shri Brahmananda Sarasvati). Fundamentals of Yoga. New York: Julian Press; 1959.

Nadi (yoga). Wikipedia; 2017 [accessed 21 January 2018]. Available from: https://en.wikipedia.org/w/index.php?title=Nadi_(yoga)&oldid=807001665.

New York City Council. School Diversity in NYC; 2019 [accessed 30 September 2020]. Available from: https://council.nyc.gov/data/school-diversity-in-nyc/

Newberg A, Alavi A, Baime M, Pourdehnad M. Cerebral blood flow during meditation: Comparison of different cognitive tasks. European Journal of Nuclear Medicine. 2000.

Newberg A, D'Aquili E, Rause V. Why God won't go away: brain science and the biology of belief. Reprint ed. New York: Ballantine Books; 2002.

Newberg AB, Wintering N, Khalsa DS, Roggenkamp H, Waldman MR. Meditation effects on cognitive function and cerebral blood flow in subjects with memory loss: A preliminary study. Journal of Alzheimer's Disease. 2010;20(2):517–26. doi:10.3233/jad-2010-1391

Official Website of the City of New York. Mayor de Blasio Announces New York City Poverty Rate Hits Historic Low; 2019 [accessed 27 October 2020]. Available from: https://www1.nyc.gov/office-of-the-mayor/news/449-19/mayor-de-blasio-new-york-city-poverty-rate-hits-historic-low

OpenStax. Anatomy & Physiology. Chapter 15.1 Divisions of the Autonomic Nervous System. In: OpenStax CNX. 26 February 2016 [accessed 29 July 2019]. Available from: https://openstax.org/books/anatomy-and-physiology/pages/15-1-divisions-of-the-autonomic-nervous-system

Park CL, Riley KE, Bedesin E, Stewart MV. Why practice yoga? Practitioners' motivations for adopting and maintaining yoga practice. Journal of Health Psychology. 2016;21(6):887–96.

Parker S, Bharati SV, Fernandez M. Defining yoga-nidra: traditional accounts, physiological research, and future directions. International Journal of Yoga Therapy. 2013;23(1):11–16.

Patañjali. The Yoga-Sūtra of Patañjali: A new translation with commentary. (C. Hartranft, Trans.). Boston, MA: Shambhala Publications; 2003.

Pilkington K, Gerbarg P, Brown R. Yoga therapy for anxiety. In: Principles and practice of yoga in health care. 1st ed. Edinburgh: Handspring Pub Ltd.; 2016.

Poppa T, Bechara A. The somatic marker hypothesis: revisiting the role of the 'body-loop' in decision-making. Current Opinion in Behavioral Sciences. 2018; 19:61–6. https://doi.org/10.1016/j.cobeha.2017.10.007

Porges SW. Love: an emergent property of the mammalian autonomic nervous system. Psychoneuroendocrinology. 1998;23(8):837–61. doi:10.1016/s0306-4530(98)00057-2.

Porges S. How your nervous system sabatoges your ability to relate: An interview with Stephen Porges about his polyvagal theory; April 2006.

Porges S. The polyvagal theory: New insights into adaptive reactions of the autonomic nervous system. Cleveland Clinic Journal of Medicine. 2009;76(Suppl 2):S86–S90. doi: 10.3949/ccjm.76.s2.17

Porges SW. The polyvagal theory: neurophysiological foundations of emotions, attachment, communication, and self-regulation. The Norton series on interpersonal neurobiology. New York: W.W. Norton; 2011.

Porges S. Vagal pathways, portals to compassion. In: Seppala, EM, Simon-Thomas, E, et al., Oxford Handbook of Compassion Science. Oxford: Oxford University Press; 2017, pp. 187-204.

Porges SW, Dana D. Clinical applications of the polyvagal theory: The emergence of polyvagal-informed therapies. New York: W. W. Norton & Company; 2018:63.

Pozuelos JP, Mead BR, Rueda MR, Malinowski P. Short-term mindful breath awareness training improves inhibitory control and response monitoring. Progress in Brain Research Meditation. 2019;137–63. doi:10.1016/bs.pbr.2018.10.019

Pratipaksha Bhavana. Yogapedia; 2018 [accessed 22 January 2018]. Available from: https://www.yogapedia.com/definition/6192/pratipaksha-bhavana

Psychosynthesis Counselor Training Program, Synthesis Center, Amherst, MA, 1986.

Radha SS. Kundalini yoga for the West. Boulder and London: Shambala; 1978.

Raghuraj P, Telles S. Immediate effect of specific nostril manipulating yoga breathing practices on autonomic and respiratory variables. Applied Psychophysiology and Biofeedback. 2008;33(2):65–75.

Rāja yoga. Wikipedia; 2017 [accessed 20 January 2018]. Available from: https://en.wikipedia.org/w/index.php?title=R%C4%81ja_yoga&oldid=811885861.

Rama S. Enlightenment without God. Honesdale, PA: Himalayan Institute Press; 1982.

Ramanathan M, Bhavanani A. Understanding how yoga works: A short review of findings from Cyter, Pondicherry, India. European Journal of Pharmaceutical and Medical Research. 2017;4(1):256–62.

Rizzolatti G, Fogassi L, Gallese V. Mirrors in the mind. Scientific American. 2006;295(5):54–61.

Robin M. A handbook for yogasana teachers: the incorporation of neuroscience, physiology, and anatomy into the practice. Tucson, AZ: Wheatmark; 2009.

Rosenberg S. Accessing the healing power of the vagus nerve: Self-help exercises for anxiety, depression, trauma, and autism. Berkeley, CA: North Atlantic Books; 2017.

Rubia K. The neurobiology of meditation and its clinical effectiveness in psychiatric disorders. Biological Psychology. 2009;82(1):1–11.

Sannella L. The Kundalini experience: psychosis or transcendence. Integral Publishers; 1987.

Sarang PS, Telles, S. Oxygen consumption and respiration during and after two yoga relaxation techniques. Applied Psychophysiology and Biofeedback. 2006;31(2):143–53.

Saraswati SS, Hiti JK. Beyond the body and mind. In: Yoga nidra. Munger, India: Bihar School of Yoga; 1984:53–8.

Satchidānanda SS. Integral yoga hatha. New York: Holt, Rinehart, Winston; 1970.

Satchidānanda, S.S. The yoga sutras of Patanjali. Pomfret Center, CT: Integral Yoga Publications; 1978.

Satchidānanda S. The key to peace. Buckingham, VA: Integral Yoga Publications; 2011.

Satyananda yoga nidra certification course manual. Cleveland Heights, OH: Yoga Academy of North America; 2012.

Schäfer C, Rosenblum MG, Kurths J, Abel HH. Heartbeat synchronized with ventilation. Nature. 1998;392(6673): 239–40. doi: 10.1038/32567

Schauer M, Elbert T. Dissociation following traumatic stress: Etiology and treatment. Journal of Psychology. 2010;218:109127.

Schwartz A. Connection and co-regulation in psycho-therapy; 2018 [accessed 4 November 2020]. Available from: https://drarielleschwartz.com/connection-co-regu-lation-psychotherapy-dr-arielle-schwartz/#.X6LlXoj7SM9

Schwartz A. The vagus nerve in trauma recovery; 2019 [accessed 28 October 2020]. Available from: https://drari-elleschwartz.com/the-vagus-nerve-in-trauma-recovery-dr-arielle-schwartz/#.XZ-QpS2ZNQI

Self-regulation. Psychology; 2020. [accessed 28 October 2020]. Available from: https://psychology.iresearchnet.com/health-psychology-research/self-regulation/

Shankaracharya, Angot M. Taittiriya upanisad: Avec le commentaire de Samkara. Paris: Institut de civilisation indienne; 2007.

Shannahoff-Khalsa DS, Beckett LR. Clinical case report: efficacy of yogic techniques in the treatment of obsessive-compulsive disorders. The International Journal of Neu-roscience. 1996;85(1–2):1–17.

Shannahoff-Khalsa DS, Boyle MR, Buebel ME. The effects of unilateral forced nostril breathing on cognition. The International Journal of Neuroscience. 1991;57(3–4): 239–49.

Shapiro F. Eye movement desensitization and reprocess-ing (EMDR) therapy: Basic principles, protocols, and procedures. New York: The Guilford Press; 2018.

Shea MJ. The multivagal safety system. Unpublished chart; n.d. Sherin JE, Nemeroff CB. Post-traumatic stress disor-der: the neurobiological impact of psychological trauma. Dialogues in Clinical Neuroscience. 2011;13(3):263–78.

Shields RW. Heart rate variability with deep breathing as a clinical test of cardiovagal function. Cleveland Clinic Journal of Medicine 2009;76(suppl 2):S37–S40.

Siegel DJ. The developing mind: How relationships and the brain interact to shape who we are. New York: Guilford Press; 1999.

Siegel DJ. An interpersonal neurobiology approach to psychotherapy. Psychiatric Annals. 2006;36(4): 248–56.

Siegel DJ. The mindful brain: reflection and attunement in the cultivation of well-being. 1st ed. New York: W. W. Norton & Company; 2007.

Siegel, Dan: inspire to rewire; 2018 [accessed 21 January 2018]. Available from: http://www.drdansiegel.com/.

Siegel, D.J. inspire to rewire, https://www.psychologytoday.com/intl/blog/inspire-rewire

Sivananda SS. Thought power. 6th ed. Tehri-Garhwal, India: Divine Life Society; 1980.

Sivananda SS. Concentration and meditation. Tehri-Garhwal, India: Divine Life Society; 2009.

Sivananda S. Mantra yoga sadhana. The Divine Life Society. 2020a [accessed 11 November 2020]. Available from: http://www.sivanandaonline.org/public_html/?cmd=displaysection&section_id=525

Sivananda S. What is this ego? The Divine Life Society. 2020b [accessed 13 November 2020]. Available from: https://www.sivanandaonline.org/public_html/?cmd=dis playsection&section_id=817

Somatic therapy. Psychology Today; 2018 [accessed 28 January 2018]. Available from: https://www.psychologytoday.com/therapy-types/somatic-therapy.

Soos MP, McComb D. Sinus Arrhythmia. Treasure Island, FL: StatPearls Publishing; 2020.

Staal A. Stress, cognition, and human performance: a literature review and conceptual framework. Ames Research Center, CA: NASA/TM—2004—212824; 2004.

Stableford S, Mettger W. Plain language: a strategic response to the health literacy challenge. Journal of Public Health Policy. 2007;28(1):71–93. doi:10.1057/palgrave.jphp.3200102.

Stangor C, Walinga J. Chapter 4.2: Our Brains control our thoughts, feelings, and behavior. In: Introduction to Psychology – 1st Canadian Edition. Victoria, BC: BCcampus; 2014 [accessed 29 July 2019]. Available from: https://opentextbc

Substance Abuse and Mental Health Services Administration. Trauma-informed care in behavioral health services. Treatment improvement protocol (TIP) Series 57. HHS Publication No. (SMA) 13-4801. Rockville, MD: Substance Abuse and Mental Health Services Administration; 2014.

Sue, DW. Racial microaggressions in everyday life. Psychology Today; 2010 [accessed 28 October 2020]. Available from: https://www.psychologytoday.com/us/blog/microaggressions-in-everyday-life/201010/racial-microaggressions-in-everyday-life

Sullivan M. Understanding yoga therapy. Applied philosophy and science for health and well-being. Routledge, New York; 2020.

Sullivan MB, Erb M, Schmalzl L, Moonaz S, Taylor JN, Porges SW. Yoga therapy and polyvagal theory: The convergence of traditional wisdom and contemporary neuroscience for self-regulation and resilience. Frontiers in Human Neuroscience, 2018;12. doi:10.3389/fnhum.2018.00067.

Swara yoga. – Definition from Yogapedia. (n.d.) [accessed 2 Aug. 2019]. Available from: https://www.yogapedia.com/definition/6276/swara-yoga

Telles S, Nagarathna R, Nagendra HR. Breathing through a particular nostril can alter metabolism and autonomic activities. Indian Journal of Physiology and Pharmacology. 1994;38(2):133–7.

Telles S, Reddy SK, Nagendra HR. Oxygen consumption and respiration following two yoga relaxation techniques. Applied Psychophysiology and Biofeedback. 2000;25(4):221–7.

Telles S, Yadav A, Kumar N, Sharma S, Visweswaraiah NK, Balkrishna A. Blood pressure and purdue pegboard scores in individuals with hypertension after alternate nostril breathing, breath awareness, and no intervention. Medical Science Monitor : International Medical Journal of Experimental and Clinical Research. 2013;19:61–6.

Thomas CW. Post-traumatic stress disorder: review of DSM criteria and functional neuroanatomy. Marshall Journal of Medicine. 2018;4(2): Article 6. doi: http://dx.doi.org/10.18590/mjm.2018.vol4.iss2.6

Trungpa C. Shambhala: the sacred path of the warrior. Reissue ed. Boston, MA; Enfield: Shambhala; 2007.

Tsur N, Defrin R, Lahav Y, Solomon Z. The traumatized body: Long-term PTSD and its implications for the orientation towards bodily signals. Psychiatry Research. 2018; 261:281–9. doi: 10.1016/j.psychres.2017.12.083

Tyagi A, Cohen M. Yoga and heart rate variability: A comprehensive review of the literature. International Journal of Yoga. 2016;9(2):97–113. doi: 10.4103/0973-6131.183712

Uebelacker L, Lavretsky H, Tremont G. Yoga therapy for depression. In: Principles and practice of yoga in health care, 1st ed. Edinburgh: Handspring Publishing Ltd.; 2016.

Vahia NS, Doongaji D, Jeste D, Kapoor S, Ardhapurkar I, Ravindranath S. Further experience with the therapy based upon concepts of patanjali in the treatment of psychiatric disorders. Indian Journal of Psychiatry. 1973;15:32–7.

Vaish A, Grossmann T, Woodward A. Not all emotions are created equal: The negativity bias in social-emotional development. Psychological Bulletin. 2008;134(3):383–403.

Van Buren BR, Weierich MR. Peritraumatic tonic immobility and trauma-related symptoms in adult survivors of childhood sexual abuse: The role of post-trauma cognitions. Journal of Child Sexual Abuse. 2015;24(8):959–74. doi: 10.1080/10538712.2015.1082003

van der Kolk BA. The body keeps the score: brain, mind, and body in the healing of trauma. New York: Viking; 2014.

van der Kolk BA, Stone L, West J, Rhodes A, Emerson D, Suvak M, Spinazzola J. Yoga as an adjunctive treatment for posttraumatic stress disorder: a randomized controlled trial. Journal of Clinical Psychiatry. 2014;75(6):e559–65.

Weintraub A. Bee Breath (Brahmari) Practice. Lifeforce Yoga; 2014 [accessed 29 October 2020]. Available from: https://yogafordepression.com/bee-breath-brahmari-practice/

Weitzberg E, Lundberg JO. Humming greatly increases nasal nitric oxide. American Journal of Respiratory Critical Care Medicine. 2002;166(2):144–5.

Werntz DA, Bickford RG, Bloom FE, Shannahoff-Khalsa DS. Alternating cerebral hemispheric activity and the lateralization of autonomic nervous function. Human Neurobiology. 1983;2(1):39–43.

Winblad NE, Changaris M, Stein PK. Effect of somatic experiencing resiliency-based trauma treatment training on quality of life and psychological health as potential markers of resilience in treating professionals. Frontiers in Neuroscience. 2018;12:70. doi:10.3389/fnins.2018.00070

Winerman L. The mind's mirror. American Psychological Association; 2005 [accessed 21 January 2018]. Available from: http://www.apa.org/monitor/oct05/mirror.aspx

World Health Organization. Draft of 11th edition of the International Classification of Disease. 2018 [accessed 29 October 2020]. Available from: https://www.who.int/classifications/icd/en/

Yoga Journal editors. Deepak Chopra's 7 spiritual laws of yoga challenge: day 1. Yoga Journal. 2018 [accessed 11 November 2020]. Available from: https://www.yogajournal.com/yoga-101/deepak-chopra-7-spiritual-laws-yoga-challenge-day-1

Yoon S, Zuccarello M, Rapoport RM. PCO_2 and pH regulation of cerebral blood flow. Frontiers in Physiology. 2012;3:365. doi:10.3389/fphys.2012.00365

Zelano C, Jiang H, Zhou G, Arora N, Schuele S, Rosenow J, Gottfried JA. Nasal respiration entrains human limbic oscillations and modulates cognitive function. Journal of Neuroscience. 2016;36(49):12448–67.

Zhou S, Hur K, Shen J, Wrobel B. Impact of sinonasal disease on depression, sleep duration, and productivity among adults in the United States. Laryngoscope Investigative Otolaryngology. 2017;2(5):288–94. doi:10.1002/lio2.87

Zimmer HR, Campbell J. Philosophies of India. Delhi: Motilal Banarsidass; 1990.